Counseling Anxiety and Depression in Adolescents

Jagruti Sundaram

Copyright © 2023 by Jagruti Sundaram
All rights reserved.

CONTENTS

S.NO.	CHAPTERS	PAGE NO.
Chapter – 1	**Introduction**	**1-50**
	❖ Anxiety	1
	❖ Theories of anxiety	5
	❖ Depression	8
	❖ Features of Depression	12
	❖ Theories of Depression	16
	❖ Interventions	22
	❖ Defining Adolescence	29
	❖ Theories of Adolescence	33
	❖ Developmental issues in Adolescence	39
	❖ Anxiety, Depression and Adolescence	41
Chapter – 2	**Review of Literature**	**51-109**
	❖ Anxiety and Counseling	51
	❖ Depression, Anxiety and Optimism	55
	❖ Depression and Counseling	59
	❖ Depression, Anxiety and Rumination	68
	❖ Effectiveness of Group Counseling	81
	❖ School-based Interventions	98
Chapter – 3	**Methodology**	**110 - 162**
	❖ Rationale	110
	❖ Objectives	110
	❖ Hypotheses	112
	❖ Variables	114
	❖ Research design	114
	❖ Sample	115
	❖ Measures	116
	❖ Procedure	126
	❖ Description of Group Counseling Program	127
	❖ Statistical analysis	162

Chapter – 4	**Results and Discussion**	**163 - 184**
	❖ Section 1 - Descriptive Statistics	
	❖ Section 2 - Experimental and Control Group pre-test comparisons	
	❖ Section 3 – Experimental and Control Group post-test comparisons	
	❖ Section 4 – Experimental group pre-post-test comparisons	
	❖ Section 5 – Control group pre-post-test comparison	
Chapter – 5	**Summary, Major Findings, Conclusion, Limitations Implications and Recommendations for Future Research**	**185-193**
		194-251

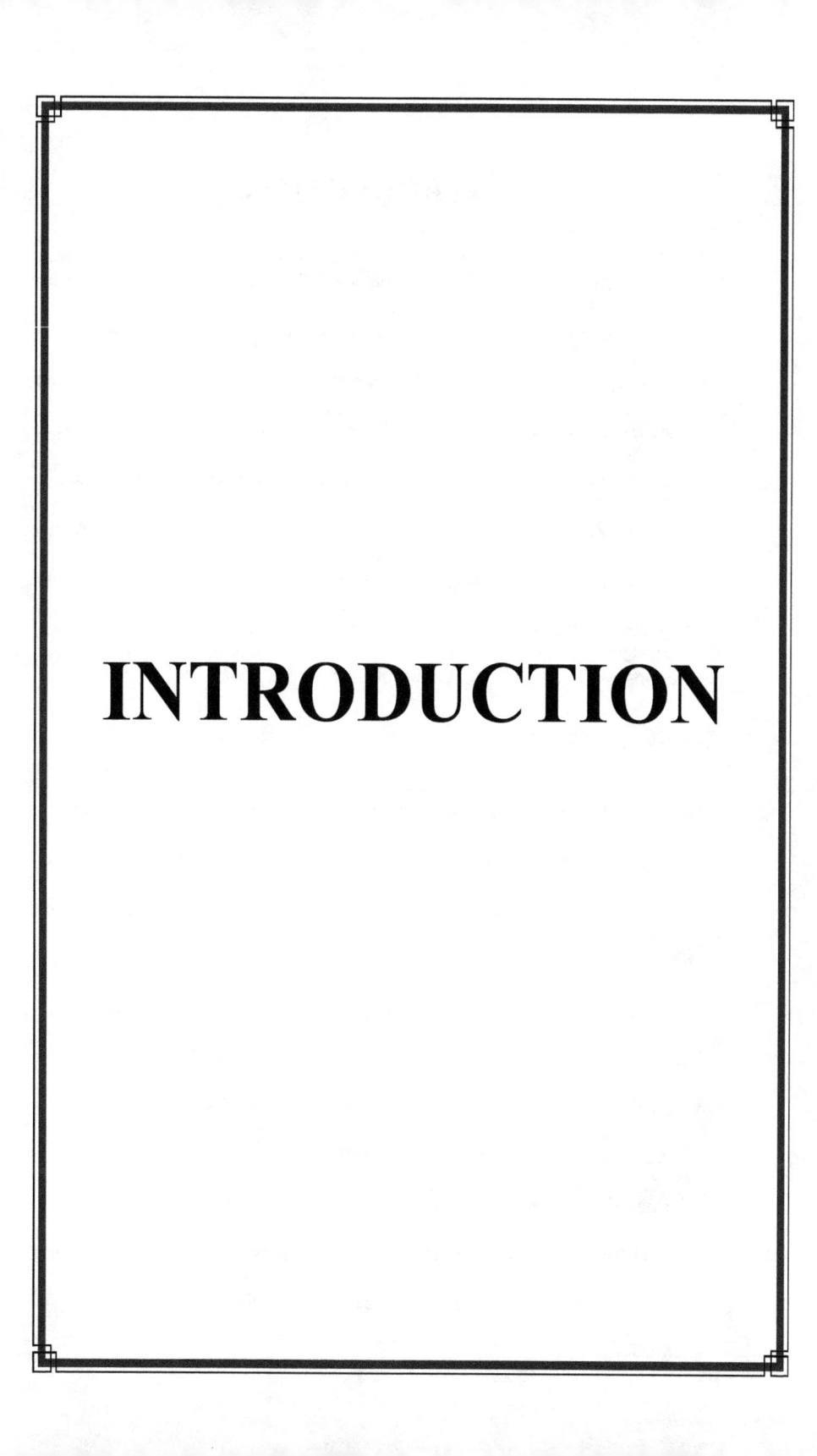

INTRODUCTION

INTRODUCTION

In the modern complex societies, which are full of stresses and strains, almost everybody experiences feelings of depression at one time or another. The emotions of feeling sad, unhappy or disappointed are a part of a human being's normal existence and are experienced by everyone almost on a daily basis. Such emotions may be associated with failure in academics, setback in a relationship, loss in a financial investment, breakup of a love affair, or with the death of a loved one. However, after feeling low for a few days, during which time there can be changes in the sleep pattern and appetite, disinterest in daily chores etc., the person undergoing depressive symptoms usually returns to normal within a reasonable period of time.

ANXIETY

Anxiety can be studied in a categorical way (diagnosis: yes or no), or in a dimensional way (symptom or severity scores). While in the past the categorical approach dominated, in recent years, increasing attention has been given to anxiety symptoms which do not meet diagnostic criteria. Due to the large variety in definitions and assessment methods of anxiety symptoms, it is difficult to estimate their prevalence. Anxiety symptoms predict the onset of anxiety disorder and depression, and have been associated with lower levels of well-being even before they reach disorder status. Hence, it is important to assess anxiety symptoms across adolescence in order to recognize potential anxiety problems and prevent the development of anxiety disorders. By merely focusing on anxiety disorders, we would disregard warning signs and an opportunity for prevention and early intervention.

In this thesis, I focus on factors that are associated with anxiety symptoms in adolescence in order to better help understand potential risk factors and outcomes of anxiety symptoms. In this chapter, I will introduce the research themes of the thesis. Proper measurement of anxiety symptoms in longitudinal studies Longitudinal studies are an invaluable tool for tracking the development of anxiety symptoms. To study the development of anxiety, anxiety needs to be measured repeatedly over time in the same individuals. In doing so, it is tempting to assume that any change we measure with our instrument reflects true and potentially meaningful changes in the anxiety symptom levels. However, for this assumption to be true, it first needs to be established that the instrument measures anxiety symptoms similarly at different ages across adolescence - a feature called longitudinal measurement invariance.

An instrument can be tested for its measurement invariance properties with a hierarchical set of psychometric tests. If longitudinal measurement invariance has been established, we can assume that a change in measured anxiety severity reflects a true change in the anxiety level across time; whereas if longitudinal measurement invariance criteria are not being met, a change in assessed anxiety symptom levels over time may reflect differences in measurement sensitivity across time rather than a true change in anxiety levels. Most importantly, if measurement invariance has not been established in an instrument, we simply cannot tell how much our findings can be trusted. Hence, it is important to first establish the measurement invariance properties of an instrument, so that the level of longitudinal measurement invariance can be taken into account when interpreting change or stability of anxiety symptom levels across time.

A developmental process that coincides with adolescence is puberty. Puberty is a period during which extensive physical development occurs, including physical growth and the development of primary and secondary sexual characteristics. Along with these physical changes, social and emotional changes occur. Most research on puberty has focused on the level of physical development, which can be assessed by determining the pubertal status through questions or examination of the occurrence of physical changes that typically happen during puberty. Findings from studies assessing the association between anxiety symptoms and pubertal status are mixed: some found either a lack of association, or state anxiety to be higher at early stages of pubertal development , while studies assessing anxiety subtypes found symptoms to positively correlate with pubertal status . In summary, previous studies carefully suggest that advanced pubertal status is associated with a higher likelihood of anxiety symptoms, which cannot merely be explained by increasing chronological age .More recently, studies have focused on pubertal timing as a potentially significant factor when assessing anxiety symptoms. Pubertal timing refers to the timing of when pubertal development occurs in relation to peers, i.e. it relates whether an adolescent is ahead of peers in pubertal development (early pubertal timing), in line with peers (on-time) or behind peers in pubertal development (late pubertal timing). Notably, while pubertal status is of influence when determining pubertal timing, it is mostly the peer reference group that determines pubertal timing, e.g. early pubertal timing can refer to almost any pubertal developmental stage. Therefore, pubertal timing is closely related to the social component of pubertal development.

Adolescents who are ahead of peers in pubertal development may experience the biological, psychological and social challenges associated with puberty before they may be psychologically prepared to cope with them effectively, which can be a risk factor for anxiety symptoms and disorders. Studies investigating the association between pubertal timing and anxiety symptoms have found mixed support for the theory that early developers have more anxiety symptoms, with several studies supporting this theory, while others finding conditional support, or no support. These inconsistencies in findings spur new approaches to better understand this association.

In most of the studies, pubertal timing was determined once. The implicit assumption is that pubertal timing does not change across puberty. However, studies have shown that adolescents go through puberty at a different tempo, so that an adolescent who is "late" in pubertal timing at one point may "catch up" and be "on-time" at a later point. Yet, so far merely one study has explicitly adopted this dynamic approach: Reynolds and Juvonen allowed for intraperson variability when they assessed pubertal timing six times across a three year period. Indeed, they found pubertal timing to be a dynamic concept, with on average 18% of their sample changing in pubertal timing between assessment waves.

A related issue concerns the assumption that the association between pubertal timing and anxiety symptoms is constant across all of adolescence. The study by Reynolds and Juvonen was the first to explicitly consider and confirm that the association between pubertal timing and social anxiety symptoms probably depends on age across adolescence. Both the dynamic approach to pubertal timing and an age-varying approach to the association between pubertal timing and anxiety symptoms are new and important domains to explore as they may contribute to a better understanding of individuals at risk for anxiety symptoms. The relationship between the development of depression and anxiety within an adolescent population is a promising area of inquiry. The increase in sub-clinical levels of anxiety and depression, where symptoms are present but do not meet criteria for a depressive or anxiety disorder, has been linked to developmental changes in adolescence.

Defining what is normal and abnormal adolescent behaviour is not a simple task for researchers. Most would agree that there is an array of factors that contribute to normal and abnormal behavior (Santrock, 2001; Ingram & Price, 2001). The field of developmental psychopathology has largely focused on identifying, exploring, and confirming developmental pathways of adolescent problems and disorders. Conceptualizing the relationship between risk factors of particular disorders in adolescents holds implications for ways in which these individuals may be aided in adapting and coping with adulthood.

Theories of Anxiety

Keeping in mind that explanations of anxiety have for centuries been derived from theories and models popular at the current time. Humans have always accepted that behaviours or traits can be caused by outside entities. The supernatural model was the accepted theory of understanding psychopathology for much of our recorded history (Barlow & Durand, 2005). Through the lens of this model, unexplained and irrational behaviour was often seen as a sign of evil. During the 14th and 15th century, insanity was believed to be a natural phenomenon caused by mental or emotional stress (Barlow & Durand, 2005). Mental anxiety and depression were recognized as an illness caused by demonic influence, but they were seen as curable. Treatments at this time included exorcism, bloodletting and some more humane treatments like ointments or baths (Barlow & Durand, 2005). From a historical perspective, anxiety and depression have shared symptoms and treatments dating back to the 14th century.

To date, varying theories account for the etiology of anxiety. Consistent with the diathesis-stress model of psychopathology, anxiety has been attributed to neurochemical (Gray & McNaughton, 1995) and genetic factors (Turner, Beidal, & Costello, 1987), which in combination with life stressors significantly increase vulnerability to the disorder. Turner et al. (1987) found that children who had parents with anxiety disorders were more likely to be anxious, report school difficulties, worry about family members and themselves, exhibit somatic complaints, and spend time alone compared to the control groups. Barret (2000) also outlines important developmental factors that are especially salient to the study of adolescent anxiety. First, infant temperament can predict later anxiety, which seems to support the presence of a biological vulnerability, and when combined with insecure attachment, the risks are heightened. Early experiences with uncontrollability, which can be due, in part, to overly controlling parenting, can also lead to increased anxiety (Barlow et al., 1996). In adolescence, when abstract reasoning increases and peers become more influential than parents, fear of negative evaluation, fear about future, and social fears develop (Barret, 2000).

Anxiety disorders are among the most prevalent diagnosis within the United States and they are the most common type of mental disorder found in adolescents (Kasahni & Orvaschel, 1988). Prevalence rates for anxiety in a community sample of adolescents vary considerably. Depending on the specifics of methods, stringency of diagnostic criteria, and other particularities of a study, clinical anxiety disorders have been estimated to occur in 5.7% to 28.8% of community adolescents (Costello & Angold, 1995; Essau, Conradt & Petermann, 2000; Kashani & Orvascal, 1988; Lewinsohn et al. 1993; Verhulst, van der Ende, Ferninand & Kasius, 1997; Woodward & Fergusson, 2001). According to the Canadian and Community Health Survey, 2.3% of adolescents and young adults (age 15 to 24) have had panic disorder, 0.8% agoraphobia, and 4.8% social phobia (Statistics Canada, 2002). Other studies report lifetime prevalence rates for anxiety disorders in community samples of adolescents ranging from 9.15 to 18.60% (Lewinsohn et al., 1993; Essau et al., 2000). More specifically, panic disorder ranged from 0.50 to 1.19%, agoraphobia from 0.60 to 4.10%, social phobia from 1.46 to 1.60%, specific phobia from 2.12 to 3.50%, and obsessive-compulsive disorder from 0.6 to 1.3%.

One possible source of discrepancy between studies is the diagnostic criteria used. While it is important to know the estimated number of adolescents who do meet criteria for a clinically diagnosable disorder, it also seems that this information does not provide a complete picture of the anxiety experienced by this population. Few studies have examined the prevalence of sub-clinical anxiety symptoms in adolescents, despite findings suggesting that sub-clinical levels of anxiety can also cause considerable levels of distress.

The onset of some types of anxiety disorder tends to be in early adulthood, whereas others tend to emerge in childhood or adolescence. Parallel with the literature on the prevalence of anxiety disorders, onset typically occurs in adolescence (Dozois & Dobson, 2004). This finding highlights the importance of identifying early indicators of anxiety within this population due to the fact that many adolescents experience mild to moderate (sub-clinical) levels of anxiety. Consequently, sub-clinical levels of anxiety in adolescents may have adverse affects on development (Ohannessian et al., 1996).

Unfortunately, compared to the empirically-based knowledge about depression, knowledge about adolescent anxiety is less available, perhaps because anxiety, specifically as a research focus, has been largely neglected (Ohannessian et al., 1999).

DEPRESSION

"I am depression.
Cold like arctic mist, I dampen your spirit and your soul.
I fill your thoughts with gloom.
When I am with you, you are but a withered leaf beneath wet snow with nowhere to go.
Still, I can do much more. I can fill your mind with graveyard thoughts and make you teary.

Knaus, 2006

Depression is a state of sadness that has advanced to the point of being disruptive to an individual's social functioning and daily activities requiring clinical intervention. "Depression" comes from the latin word *depressio*, meaning to press down. Many researchers assume that the term "depression" refers not simply to a state of depressed mood, but to a syndrome comprising mood disorder, psychomotor changes and a variety of somatic disturbances.

Depression is a psychological condition that changes how we think and feel and also affects our social behaviour and sense of physical well being. When mired in depression, happiness eludes us. Pleasure is nowhere to be found. Our ambitions clot. Our strength leaves us. We worry. We lack confidence. We think we are unloved. Our thoughts are filled with cries of helplessness and hopelessness. We feel trapped. Our attention is adrift. Our relationships sour. We feel stuck, numbed, dull and lifeless. Encapsulated within a persistently negative mood, gloom seems impenetrable. Interests are dampened. This process practically always include patterns of negative, depressive thoughts including helplessness, hopelessness and worthlessness (Knaus, 2006).

This painful process of depression can start with an overwhelming trauma or slowly build from a long history of stress and negative thinking or a family history of depression and negative life circumstances. Depression can be viewed as a persistent and recurring scourge that can involve multiple coexisting conditions such as anxiety and anger (Pettit & Joiner, 2006). This condition is clearly an equal opportunity disability that can affect anyone at any economic level, from childhood to old age. Kessler et al. (2003) found that approximately 16% of adults will experience depression in their lifetime. Depression is the most commonly encountered disorder among psychiatric outpatients (45%) and only 31% of depression sufferers are suffering from depression alone (Zimmerman et al., 2008).

In India, depression is a major public health problem resulting in increased suffering, diminished social and occupational functioning as well as high levels of suicide. A number of Indian studies (Amin et al., 1998; Nambi et al., 2002; Pothen et al., 2003) have reported a wide range of prevalence of depression in India. A World Health Organization study examining 15 primary care centers, in 14 countries worldwide, including Bangalore in Southern India, was conducted to assess psychological problems in general healthcare on the basis of which it was determined that 9.1% of the general population in Bangalore, India suffers from depression (Goldberg and

Lecruiber, 1995). Patel (1996) found that 40% of Indian adults attending primary health care clinics were depressed. Nandi et al. (2000) suggested that the rate of depression has increased significantly over the years in India as well. Madhav (2001) found that a prevalence rate for depression in India is 31.2 per 1000 population. Sengupta (2005) stated that depression is a major health problem in countries like India. Poongothai et al. (2009) in the largest population based study from India reported that prevalence of depression among south Indians is 15.1%. This is consistent with the figures reported for developing countries (10-44%) by WHO (2001).

Tsui (2008) reported that the National Institute of Mental Health and Neuro-Sciences (NIMHANS), Bangalore, India, found that 1 in every 15 adult Indians suffers from depressive illness. At least 10% of the population suffers from depression that needs professional and medical help and as much as 40 per cent of the population is demoralized and likely to cross the line to clinical depression sometime. Reddy (2010) stated that Indian union health ministry estimates state that 120,000 people commit suicide every year in India and that majority of those committing suicide suffer from depression. A review of eight epidemiological studies on depression in South Asia shows that the prevalence in primary care was 26.3%. In the Goa study, the rate of depressive disorders was 46.5% in adult primary care attendees (Reddy, 2010).

Over the past several years, the prevalence of depression has been on the rise because of several reasons such as demographic shifts to urban and suburban areas and loss of small community support, rapid social and economic changes that appear outside the scope of individual control, sedentary lifestyles and earlier pubescence. More than a dozen epidemiologic studies around the world have presented data suggesting that depression has become more common and has been on the rise in the last half century (Ballenger et al., 2001; Kessler et al., 2005).

According to World Health Organization, clinical depression which is currently the fourth leading illness, worldwide, is expected to become the second leading cause of disability by the year 2020 (Murray and Lopez, 1997; World Health Organisation, 2002). Cipriani et al. (2009) suggested that depression is expected to show a rising trend over the next twenty years.

Major depression is a common, costly, disabling and one of the most burdensome disorders worldwide (Grant et al., 2004; Olsen et al., 2004; Donohue and Pincus, 2007). Major depressive disorder is associated with grave consequences in terms of excessive mortality, morbidity, loss of productivity, income, poor health and suicide. Several researchers have found that the relationship between depression and mortality has been on the rise for the past few years (Vinkers et al., 2004; Adamson et al., 2005; Wulsin et al., 2005).

Depression carries a high mortality rate because it is a risk factor for many major disease related causes of death as well as suicide (Mykletun et al., 2007). In India 2% of those who commit suicide suffer from major depressive disorder (Manoranjanjitham et al., 2010). Depression is associated with higher morbidity (Kessler et al., 2003). Murray & Lopez (1996) in The Global Burden of Disease Study report that major depression costs three times more than the price of alcohol abuse. Depression is associated with increased rates of chronic illness, health care utilizations and absenteeism at work (Stewart et al., 2003; Stein et al., 2006; Greenberg et al., 2006a). In the year 2000, the estimated cost of depression due to personal impairment, medical costs and low productivity was $83.1 billion (Greenberg et al., 2003). Depression is expected to overtake heart disease as the largest killer by 2020 and is now the largest cause of absenteeism in businesses costing over $ 51 billion a year in productivity (Grimes, 2009).

FEATURES OF DEPRESSION

Major depressive disorder is diagnosed based on the presence of a constellation of signs and symptoms that are characteristic of the illness. DeRubies et al. (2008) stated that depression can be defined as both a syndrome and a disorder. As a syndrome it involves episodes of sadness, loss of interest, pessimism, negative beliefs about the self, decreased motivation, behavioural passivity, changes in sleep, appetite and sexual interest and suicidal thoughts and impulses. Baghai et al. (2008) stated that the core symptoms of depression are a combination of psychological and somatic symptoms, often combined with psychomotor and cognitive disturbances.

Deb and Bhattacharjee (2009) stated that the term 'depression' is used to describe a range of experiences from a slightly noticeable and temporary mood decrease to a profoundly impaired and even life-threatening disorder. Basically depression refers to a constellation of experiences including not only mood but also physical, mental and behavioural experiences that define more prolonged impairing and severe conditions that may be clinically diagnosable as the syndrome of depression.

Major depressive disorder (MDD) is characterized by one or more major depressive episodes and the absence of manic episodes. A major depressive episode is defined by depressive mood or loss of interest or pleasure in almost all usual activities accompanied by other depressive symptoms. DSM-IV-TR (American Psychiatric Association, 2000) specifies that at least five of nine specific depressive symptoms (e.g. depressed mood most of the day, diminished interest in nearly all activities, significant weight loss or weight gain, insomia or hypersomia, lethargy, fatigue, indecisiveness, feelings of guilt and thoughts of death) must be present nearly every day for at least two weeks to make a diagnosis of major depressive disorder and that the symptoms must cause clinically significant distress or impairment in social, occupational, or other important areas of functioning. Somatic symptoms are common in patients with depression (Tylee and Gandhi, 2005; Demyttenaere et al., 2006), including fatigue and lack of energy (Baldwin and Papakostas, 2006) and painful physical symptoms such as headaches and back pain (Currie and Wang, 2004). Perlis (2005) suggested that DSM-IV does not include irritability as a symptom of major depressive disorder among adults, despite the fact that irritability is commonly found in clinical samples of adults with depression. Feixas et al. (2008) found that those with depressive disorders perceived themselves and others more negatively, perceived themselves as different from others and generated fewer constructs to describe self and others in comparison to the non-clinical group. Bjarehed et al. (2010) reported that reduced anticipation of future positive events is a defining characteristic of depression.

According to an analysis of data from the World Health Organisation, 69% of patients in primary care settings meeting the DSM-IV/ICD-10 criteria for depression presented somatic symptoms as their primary reason for seeking medical care (Simon et al., 1999).

The term depression encompasses a variety of conditions that differ in severity. The DSM-IV recognizes the clinical utility of distinguishing levels of severity by including a dimensional severity specified that is based on a combination of number of symptoms, degree of functional impairment and presence of psychotic symptoms. Although severity alone is insufficient for an adequate classification of depression, it is an important part of classification system because it has significant implications for treatment, prognosis and etiology. Discussions of dimensional models of depression have almost always focused exclusively on variations in symptom severity (Andrews et al., 2007). Depression can range in severity from mild disruptions of normal mood to disorders of psychotic intensity. Major depression can be categorized into mild, moderate and severe depression.

Mild depression ranges from a threshold number of symptoms (4-5) with minimal functional impairment. While symptoms are usually less severe and less numerous in mild depression than moderate and severe depression, they still have the ability to cause disruption and distress. Mild depression causes an impact upon our daily activities. The sufferer shows a diminished interest in things which he or she usually finds interesting or enjoyable. The sufferer may carry on with their normal lives, only appearing low in spirits and possibly less sharp in their thinking or in their interest. They may stop doing things they do not actually have to do, but will often continue with essentials, such as going to work or caring for the family. However, they will tend not to be as conscientious about these things as previously, or will become upset because they feel they are not coping as well as they should because they feel too tired.

Moderate Depression is characterized by the presence of 5-6 symptoms including 2 key symptoms (i.e. persistent sadness, loss of interest or low energy). Moderate depression fits somewhere between mild and severe depression. The characteristics of moderate depression tend to be more prominent and more enduring than those described for mild depression and less severe than those experienced in severe depression. People who experience moderate depression may find they have a reduced interest in normally pleasurable activities and simple things require real effort or just get neglected. Moderate depression can cause serious difficulties with social, work and domestic activities and if left untreated may lead to severe depression. Moderate depression usually results in a detectable reduction in self confidence or self esteem which may result in people becoming less motivated and less productive. Such people often start to worry about things unnecessarily, such as performance at work, even if they are managing to maintain their previous standards. They may be more sensitive and susceptible to feeling hurt or offended within personal relationships.

The patient's appearance is characteristic. Dress and grooming may be neglected. The facial features are characterized by a turning downwards of the corners of the mouth and by vertical furrowing of the center of the brow. The rate of blinking may be reduced. The shoulders are bent and the head is inclined forward so that the direction of the gaze is downwards. Gestural movements are reduced. It is important to note that some patients maintain a smiling exterior despite deep feelings of depression. Severe depression is characterized by the presence of all or nearly all DSM-IV depressive symptoms to a clinically severe degree and marked functional impairment in all areas of life (Anderson and Lambert, 2001). Severe depression may include extreme feelings of depression, distress, agitation and guilt. It is unlikely that the person will be able to continue with work, social and domestic activities.

Behaviour Theory of Depression

Behaviour theory by Ferster (1973, 1974) argued that depression could be equated with a state of extinction from positive reinforcement that is a state in which the person's responses no longer produce positive reinforcement. One problem that can lead to low rate of positive reinforcement is a deficit in social skills or major environmental factors.

In a theory much in line with Freud's theory of nurturing, many behaviorists believe that some individuals develop depression because they were overprotected when they were younger (Wetzel, 1984). The pressures and stressors of life out in the "real world" are just too much for them to handle. They have been taught by their parents to be passive because there was always someone looking out for them. The stressors mount and they feel inferior because they believe they are incapable of fending for themselves.

In 1974, Lewinsohn proposed a behavioural and interpersonal model of depression. Lewinsohn (1974, 1981) elaborated on this model and proposed that depression can be elicited when a person's behaviour no longer brings the accustomed reinforcement or gratification. The failure to receive positive reinforcement contingent on one's responses or an increase in the rate of negative reinforcements, in turn leads to a reduction in effort and activity, thus resulting in even less chance of coping with aversive conditions and achieving need gratification. According to Lewinsohn, depressed individuals do not receive enough positive support from significant others because they lack the social skills necessary for eliciting positive responses. Furthermore, depressed people are seen as less able of giving back to others, also thereby decreasing their chances for receiving support. The theory also hypothesizes that the maintenance of depression is influenced by the depressed individual's tendency to withdraw from social activities and therefore experience less pleasure.

Interpersonal Theory of Depression

The interpersonal theory of depression takes into account aspects of an individual's social functioning and environment. The researchers of Interpersonal Theory, Weissman and Paykel in 1974, published an innovative study on the interpersonal and personal lives of depressed women. The empirically validated interpersonal psychotherapy (IPT) was developed from their findings. However, their theory remained largely based on the broad idea that understanding and renegotiating interpersonal relationships is essential in the treatment of depression. Specific maintaining factors were not identified or tested through research.

In 1976, Coyne introduced his Interpersonal Theory of Depression which proposed that initially non-depressed but mildly dysphoric individuals seek constant excessive reassurance from others to alleviate their doubts as to their own worth and others' love for them (Coyne, 1976). Significant others often respond with reassurance, but with little success, because the potentially depressed person doubts and rejects the reassurance. As the pattern continues, the depressed person's significant others become increasingly frustrated and irritated and more likely to reject the depressed individual which is the individual's greatest fear. This rejection, in turn, exacerbates or maintains the depressed person's symptoms (Coyne, 1976).

Cognitive Theory of Depression

In the early 1970s, when cognitive psychology was becoming more mainstream, many clinical theorists shifted from a motivational-affective perspective to a cognitive approach for the study of psychopathology (Alloy et al., 1985). More specifically, much theorizing about psychopathological individuals' dysfunctional cognitive processes occurred within the area of depression. Two leading cognitive etiological theories of depression emerged during this time and continue to have great influence today. These were the Beck's cognitive model of depression (Beck, 1967, 1976; Beck et al., 1979) and reformulated learned helplessness theory of depression (Abramson et al., 1978). Both models could be described as cognitive diathesis-stress models of depression in which individuals with particular cognitive styles are hypothesized to be vulnerable to depression when faced with negative events. Beck's cognitive model is a cognitive-diathesis model in which three cognitive constructs are postulated to account for the development of depression when negative life events occur (Beck, 1967, 1976). These three constructs are schemata, cognitive errors and the cognitive triad. Schemata represent relatively enduring, cognitive organizing structures that direct the processing of situational information. Schemata are

hypothesized to develop through interactions with the environment and to be initially formed during childhood, reinforced by ongoing experience. According to Beck (1967), depressogenic schemata are negative in content and consist of immature and rigid attitudes concerning the self and its relation to the world. Dysfunctional schematic information processing constitutes a vulnerability factor in the development of depression. More specifically, when activated by negative life events, depressogenic schemata lead to automatic and systematic cognitive errors in the logic of depressives' thinking. In addition, Beck et al. (1979) suggested that depressed people think irrationally in areas, which he called the cognitive triad, i.e. negative thoughts about the self, negative thoughts about one's experiences and the surrounding world as well as negative thoughts about one's future.

Abramson's revised version of Seligman's original hopelessness model stated that an individual's expectation that highly desired outcomes are not likely to occur or that highly aversive outcomes are probable and that one has no power to change the probability of these outcomes - the expectation of hopelessness - is a proximal sufficient, but not a necessary, cause of depression (Abramson et al., 1985). The theory also specifies a causal chain of events that results in the expectation of hopelessness. The causal sequence begins with the occurrence of negative life events and ends with the onset of depressive symptoms. In between, Abramson argued that the expectation of hopelessness and thus, depressive symptoms are more likely to occur when negative life events are attributed to internal, stable and global factors than when they are attributed to external, unstable and specific factors. Furthermore, the onset of depression is more likely to occur when negative life events are viewed as important than when they are perceived as unimportant. Abramson hypothesized that some individuals possess a depressogenic attributional style, which consists of an overall tendency to attribute negative events to internal, stable and global factors and to view negative events as very important. Hence, people who exhibit the hypothesized depressive attributional style should have a higher probability than people who do not have this style of forming an expectation of hopelessness and thus, depressive symptoms. In this context, this cognitive style serves as a cognitive diathesis to depression. There has been much support in the adult depression literature for this model. For instance, a positive association has been found between depressive symptoms and depressive attributional style (Peterson & Seligman, 1984; Sweeney et al., 1986). Evidence for the hopelessness theory of depression has also been reported (Metalsky & Joiner, 1992; Metalsky et al., 1993).

Thus, while cognitive theorists differ in what they consider to be the critical cognitions for depression, they all assume that the depression related cognitions are causally related to depression i.e. the two most prominent cognitive theories of depression described above (Beck's cognitive model and the reformulated learned helplessness model) suggest that certain individuals exhibit enduring, trait like cognitive patterns that render them especially vulnerable to depression. Beck (1967) and Beck et al. (1979) postulates that negative expectancies about self, the world and the future lead to depression and Seligman et al. (1979) proposes that internal attributions for failure and external attributions for success can cause depressive disorders. While a number of correlational studies (e.g. Munoz et al., 1979) have provided strong support that certain kinds of cognitive changes are associated with depression, the direction of causation is left in doubt. Although it could be true, as the theorists suggest, that negative cognitions precede depression and in some way contribute to its occurance (Alloy, 2006), it isequally possible that negative conditions are a consequence of depression, that being depressed causes one to think negatively. Though numerous studies have substantiated Beck's prediction that depressed individuals are more prone to report dysfunctional attitudes (Zimmerman et al., 1986; Barnett & Gotlib, 1988) and negative thoughts (Dobson & Shaw, 1986; Kendell et al., 1989) than are non-depressed controls, such as depressotypic cognitions appear to be state-dependent i.e. elevated levels of dysfunctional attitudes and negative automatic thoughts are typically observed only during the depressive episode itself; the majority of investigations have found that the cognitions of remitted depressives, on average, to be indistinguishable from those of non-depressed controls (Dohr et al., 1989; Blackburn et al., 1990). Investigations of the reformulated learned helplessness models have reported a similar pattern; depressed individuals are more likely than non-depressed controls to attribute negative events to internal, stable and global causes (Brewin, 1985; Barnett & Gotlib, 1988), but the majority of reports have found no significant differences in negative attributional style between remitted depressives and controls (Fennell & Campbell, 1984; Dohr et al., 1989). The available evidence, then, suggests that depressive cognition may be largely a function of the depressed state itself, rather than a stable, trait like characteristic of individuals vulnerable to depression. It is, however, important to note that such findings are not entirely inconsistent with the predictions of Beck's cognitive model. In proposing the existence of maladaptive schemata, Beck proposed that such schemata may remain latent in vulnerable individuals until such time as they are activated by the occurrence of one or more negative life events (Beck, 1976, Beck et al., 1979). Monroe & Simons (1991) found that a number of attitudinal and attributional based predispositions which increase the risk of depressive reactions are typically inoperative in the course of normative information processing but becomes reactive with specific life stressful events. This view holds that people thought to be vulnerable to the onset of depression are typically indistinguishable from the general population and it is only when these individuals are confronted with certain stressors that differences between vulnerable and non-vulnerable persons emerge. For vulnerable persons, these life events can precipitate a pattern of negatively biased information processing that initiates the first cycle in a downward spiral of depression and non-vulnerable individuals react with appropriate levels of distress to the event not spiraling into depression (Metalsky et al., 1987; Segal et al., 1992). Segal & Ingram (1994) also proposed that depressive thinking patterns persist in vulnerable individuals but only become active and detectable following a triggering event. Thus, we can say that individuals at risk for depression may retain the tendency towards depression-inducing responses but this reactivity is likely to emerge only under certain conditions. Gotlib and Joorman (2010) stated that cognitive theories of depression posit that people's thoughts, inferences, attitudes and interpretation, which they attend to and recall information, can increase their risk for depression. Three mechanisms have been implicated in the relation between biased cognitive processing and the dysregulation of emotions in depression: the inhibitory processes and deficits in working memory, ruminative responses to negative mood states and events and the inability to use positive and rewarding stimuli to regulate negative mood. Thus, they concluded that depression is characterized by increased elaboration of negative information, by difficulties disengaging material and by deficits in cognitive control when processing negative information.

INTERVENTIONS FOR DEPRESSION

Depression is one of the most common and debilitating psychiatric disorder. Moussavi et al. (2007) stated that owing to its prevalence, its chronic and recurrent nature and its frequent co-morbidity with other chronic illnesses - both as a contributing factor and as a consequence - depression is considered to be the condition that is most responsible for health decrements worldwide. It is therefore, a global health priority to understand, prevent and treat depression. Lester and Howe (2008) also stated that the recognition and treatment of depression is a challenging area of clinical practice as there are many patients with various presentations and multitude of causes for distress. He viewed that there is a need to identify, treat and understand the perspectives of people with depression and provide them with effective, high quality, flexible and cost effective interventions.

Over the past fifty years, the scientific research on depression has discovered many ways to address and defeat this chronic disability. Depending upon the severity and nature of depression, there are a wide range of effective treatments available (Donohue and Pincus, 2007). There are a number of anti-depressant medication and psychotherapies that can be used to treat depression. Various studies have reported that antidepressant medication and psychotherapies are efficacious in treating moderate and severe forms of depression (American Psychiatric Association, 2000; DeRubies et al., 2005; Dimidjian et al., 2006). Some people with milder forms may do well with psychotherapy alone. Most do best with combined treatment: antidepressant medication to gain relatively quick symptom relief and psychotherapy to learn more effective ways to deal with life's problems, including depression. Taking into account, the patient's diagnosis and severity of symptoms, the therapist may prescribe antidepressant medication and/or one of the several forms of psychotherapy that have proven effective for depression. Psychological interventions for the treatment of depression which are as follows :

Psychological Interventions

Bortolotti et al. (2008) and Cuijpers et al. (2009c) found that psychological forms of interventions are quite effective and significantly linked to clinical improvement in depressive symptomatology. In the recent years, there has been an increase in attention to psychological treatments for depression, because of the demand of depressed patients and their families for non drug approaches as there is little evidence that having taken medication does anything to alter the risk factors that lead to subsequent relapse and recurrence (Kupfer, 2005) and most patients with chronic or recurrent depression are encouraged to stay on medication indefinitely (Hollon et al., 2002). Further, there is a recognized need for alternatives to medications, given their potential for side effects and some patients' preferences for non-pharmacological treatments for depression (Hollon & Shelton, 2001; van Schaik et al., 2004). And as such clinicians have welcomed the development of more systematic psychological approaches for patients who cannot be prescribed standard antidepressant drugs or who are unlikely to respond to this intervention alone. Zeiss et al. (1979) proposed that any psychological treatment that meets the following criteria should be effective in overcoming depression Therapy should begin with an elaborate, well-planned rationale. This rationale should provide initial structure that guides the patient to the belief that he or she can control his or her own behaviour and thereby, his or her depression. Therapy should provide training in skills that the patient can utilize to feel more effective in handling his or her daily life. These skills must be of significance to the patient and must fit with the rationale that has been presented. Therapy should emphasize the independent use of these skills by the patient outside of the therapy context and must provide enough structure so that the attainment of independent skill is possible for the patient. Therapy should encourage the patient's attribution that improvement in mood is caused by the patient's increased skillfulness and not by the therapist's skillfulness.

Hautzinger (2008) suggested that there are a number of structured psychological interventions that have been shown to be effective in reducing the symptoms of patients with depression, which are as follows:

(a) Psychodynamic Therapy

Psychodynamic therapy is based on the assumption that a person experiences depression as a result of unresolved, generally unconscious conflicts, often stemming from childhood. The goal of this type of therapy is for the patient to understand and cope better with these feelings by re-experiencing them through talking about them.

Psychodynamic therapy is administered over a period of three to four months, although it can last longer, even for years. Several researchers have found that psychodynamic therapy is effective in treating depression (Leichsenring, 2001; Leichsenring & Rabung, 2008).

(b) Interpersonal Therapy

Another therapy used with depressed patients is Interpersonal Therapy (IPT) which is a short-term psychotherapy, normally consisting of 12 to 16 weekly sessions. It was developed specifically for the treatment of major depression and focuses on correcting current social dysfunction. Weissman & Markowitz (1994) found that IPT focuses on factors that interfere with social relations. It is a treatment that focuses on the behaviours and social interactions a patient has with family and friends. The primary goal of this therapy is to improve communication skills and increase self-esteem during a short period of time. It usually lasts three to four months and works well for depression caused by mourning, relationship conflicts, major life events and social isolation. Craighead et al. (2002) found that IPT has been shown to be an effective treatment for major depressive disorder, equalling the effects of CBT. de Mello et al. (2005) and Parker et al. (2006) found interpersonal therapy to be effective in treating depression.

(c) Cognitive Behavioural Therapy

Still another promising psychosocial intervention is Cognitive Behavioural Therapy. Over the past 50 years, Cognitive Behavioural Therapy (CBT) has become one of the most effective mainstream psychosocial treatment for many emotional and behavioural problems. CBT is a psychotherapeutic approach, which is used by psychologists and therapists to help promote positive change in individuals, to help alleviate emotional distress and to address a myriad of psychological, social and behavioural issues. CBT aims to alleviate distress by modifying cognitive content and process, realigning thinking with reality (Longmore and Worrell, 2008). Cognitive Behavioural therapists identify and treat difficulties arising from an individual's irrational thinking, misperceptions, dysfunctional thoughts and faulty learning. CBT is based on the scientific fact that our thoughts cause our feelings and behaviours, not external things like people, situations and events. The benefit of this fact is that we can change the way we think to feel and act better even if the situation does not change. The therapy can be conducted with individuals, families or groups. CBT includes cognitive techniques as well as behavioural components. The former emphasizes on recognizing and challenging negative thoughts and maladaptive beliefs while the latter involves graded task assignments, pleasant events scheduling as well as other skills training such as relaxation skills, communication skills, assertiveness skills and problem solving skills (Soloman & Haaga, 2004).

Although, Beck developed cognitive therapy in the early 1960's as a treatment for depression, it has since been then applied to virtually every psychiatric disorder, as well as to general "problems of living". Sanderson and Mc Ginn (2001) stated that cognitive behaviour therapy has been traditionally used as a short term treatment for a wide range of emotional disorders and problems. CBT is at present a recommended treatment option for a number of mental disorders (Whittal, 2008), including depression (Beck et al., 1979; Tolin, 2010) personality disorders (Matusiewicz et al., 2010), marital distress (Epstein & Baucom, 2002), social phobia (Clark et al., 2003), obsessive-compulsive disorder (Butler et al., 2006), eating disorders (Wilson, 2005), generalized anxiety disorder (Dugas and Robichaud, 2007), panic disorder or agoraphobia (Marchand et al., 2009), bipolar disorders (Otto and Miklowitz, 2004), post-traumatic stress disorder (Bradley et al., 2005) and ADHD (Safren et al., 2005). It is also frequently used as a tool to deal with chronic pain for patients with illnesses such as rheumatoid arthritis (Backman, 2006), cancer (Magill et al., 2008) and insomia (Edinger et al., 2007). CBT is currently an integration of two originally separate theoretical approaches to understanding and treating psychological disorders: the behavioural approach and the cognitive approach (Ledley et al., 2005). The behavioural approach focuses exclusively on observable, measurable behaviour and ignores all mental events. It views that the mind is not worthy of exploration and it focuses instead on the interaction of environment and behaviour. The cognitive approach focuses on the role of mind and specifically on cognitions as determinants of feelings and behaviours.

The development of CBT took place in three stages. The first stage was the growth of behaviour therapy from 1950's to 1970's in two independent and parallel streams in the United Kingdom and United States. The British form of behaviour therapy derived its inspiration from the works of Pavlov, Watson, Hull, Wolpe and Eysenck, while in America, Skinner became the pioneer of the behaviourist movement. John. B. Watson, often considered to be the "father of behaviorism" saw behaviour change, as a function of learning via classical conditioning. He posited that even complex behaviours could be broken down into component behaviours that had all been acquired through simple learning process. There are three key elements of classical conditioning: the conditioned stimulus and response, the conditioned stimulus and the conditioned response. Watson believed that all learning (and thus, all behaviour change) occurs through this type of simple stimulus- response pairings. B.F. Skinner was another key figure in the rise of behaviourism. Skinner's theories of conditioning were more sophisticated than Watson's, they focused on operant rather than classical conditioning. In operant conditioning, stimuli are not thought of as eliciting responses. Instead, as organisms interact with their environments, they emit all sorts of responses, when the organism is rewarded for a particular response, the response is more likely to occur again as it is reinforced.

At that time, experimentally based principles of behaviour were applied to the modification of maladaptive human behaviour but slowly behavioural therapy started fading out of sight because the behavioural approach did apply to some of the problems, but all learned behaviours could not be explained through simple stimulus response association, as a result of which the clinicians became interested in the cognitive aspects. The second stage was the development of cognitive therapy which took place in the United States from the 1960's. The most influential pioneers in the development of Cognitive Therapy were Ellis (1962) and Beck (1964). Beck (1964) acknowledged that disordered cognitions are not a cause of abnormal behaviour or emotions, but rather are an intrinsic (yet alterable) element of such behaviour and emotions. If the critical cognitive components can be changed, then the behaviour and maladaptive emotions will automatically change. Thus, after much clinical observations and experimental testing, Beck (1964) developed the cognitive therapy, which was well supported by Ellis as well. The third stage was the merging of cognitive and behavioural principles and strategies into a coherent whole, resulting in the emergence of cognitive behavior therapy. CBT was developed by Aaron. T. Beck at the university of Pennsylvania in the early 1960's as a structured, short-term, present oriented psychotherapy for depression, directed towards solving current problems and modifying dysfunctional thinking and behaviour (Beck, 1964).

What is Adolescence?

Common sense is the collection of prejudices acquired by age eighteen.

— Albert Einstein

Adolescence is the period of transition between childhood to adulthood. It is a period when rapid physiological changes and demands for new social roles take place. The adolescents, due to these changes often face a number of crises and dilemmas. Adolescence is the period of development from pubescence of adulthood. It is the period when the child moves from dependency to autonomy. It is a period demanding significant adjustment to the physical and social changes which distinguish childhood behaviour from adult behaviour. The stage of puberty brings in a number of physical and physiological changes.

Adolescence is a stage when rapid changes take place. The individual's physical, mental, social, moral and spiritual outlooks undergo revolutionary changes. Such changes during adolescence are more rapid than during infancy and childhood. Due to these growths, adolescents' personality develops new dimensions. Many parents fail to assess these changes and generally show indifference because they do not like to slacken their control over their children. This attitude creates many problems for adolescent. During adolescence the individual wants to take independent decisions in various situations of his experiences. This is regarded by the elders as an act of indiscipline or of misconduct. Gradually, the adolescent starts to control his desire according to standards set by the society. He also begins to realize his social responsibilities. If he fails to attempt, he develops many defects in his personality. Hence, adolescence refers not only to biological growth, but also social growth within a cultural framework.

Puberty, this term is used to denote the point in time when an individual reaches sexual maturity and becomes capable of bearing offspring and reproducing the Puberty, then, is a much more specific term than adolescence. Pubescence, this term generally used to refer to the approximately two-year period that precedes puberty, it is the period when physiological changes that lead to the development of both primary and secondary sex characteristics take place. Pubescence, then, occurs during late childhood and early adolescence, with puberty occurring somewhat later. Pubescence refers to the relatively massive physiological changes occurring during the growth spurt that is completed in the early teen years for most girls and mid-teen years for most boys. This growth includes changes in height, weight, exercise tolerance, and, other subtle changes in physiological changes.

Adolescence is the age of stress and strains.

Age related physical changes and the resulting psychological disturbances may lead to greater maladjustment, stress and lead to depression in adolescents (Indira and Murthy, 1980, Jaiprakash and Murthy, 1981, 1982, Rangaswamy et al. 1982, Jamuna, 1984).

Death of a loved one as a stressful event is found as a precipitating cause leading to depression (Renner and Birren, 1980). Evidences also indicate relationship between somatic symptoms, depression and stress in adolescents. Depression was found to be the most significant factor in the development of somatic complaints. Studies by Rozzine (1996), Schulz and Williamson (1993), Smallegan (1989), Ramamurti (1996), Ramamurti and Jamuna (1984, 1992) reveals that stressful events are important co-factors in depression.

According to Beck (1983), Hammen, Ellicott, Gitlin and Jamison (1989) those who highly value interpersonal relationship are especially vulnerable to depression when negative life events occur within the interpersonal domain, such as rejection or loss of a loved one. They point out that stressful life events can precipitate depression in cognitively vulnerable individuals. Cohen (1995) report a relationship among stress, social support and depression. High stress and low levels of social support seem to be associated with and to predict depressive symptoms (Cohen and Wills, 1985). Paykel (1983) points out that recent life events precede depression at greater than control rate. Hawkins, Hawkins and Seeley (1993) also have found high stress as a crucial factor in high risk depressive symptomatology.

It is an intriguing developmental observation that the rates of depression increases during early adolescence (Rutter, 1986). The child's interpretation of the stressor, knowledge of coping strategies and sense of self-esteem or self efficacy may affect the level of distress experienced and thus the severity of depressive reactions.

Wolfe and Gilland (1987) conducted a study that reported relationship between measures of stress and depression in children. The sample of 102 children and adolescents were psychiatric inpatients that ranged in age for 6.5 to 16 years. The authors found moderate and significant intercorrelations between the stress and depression. Srivastava and Sinha (1989) confirmed that stressful events during life time are found to be related with the symptoms of depression. A more significant relationship between stressful events of past one year and symptoms of depression is also found. Lempers, Lempers and Netusil (1990) have reported positive relationship between family financial stress and depressive symptoms in adolescent children. In a study of the relationship of life stressors, personal and social resources and depression, Holahan and Moos (1991) found that under high stress, personal and social resources relate to future psychological health indirectly through adaptive coping strategies. Lempers and Nutusil (1990) studied the relationship among family financial stress, parent's emotional support for their children, academic achievement and depressive symptoms in a sample of 105, high school students from farm and non farm families. Results of analysis of variance indicate that parents from farm families report higher level of family financial stress and depression than parents from non farm families. Multiple regression analysis shows that family financial stress as reported by parents was strongly related to adolescent's depressive symptoms.

Theories of Adoloscence

Biological Theories:

Biological changes are the first sign of impending entrance into adolescence period by the child. These changes are so natural for parents, children, siblings, and others. Physical changes are carries with so many expectations of changes in behavior, such as acting "more grown up". It is not surprising, then, that considerable theorizing has centered on the importance of biological changes for explaining aspects of adolescence.

Hall's wrote, a monumental two-volume text entitled *Adolescence,* in 1904. Hall's thinking about psychological developmental was significantly influenced by Darwin's *On the Origin of Spices* (1985). Hall believed that the individual developed in a series of stages that corresponded to the stages passed through by mankind in its development. He reveled the fact that as the organism matured, its behavior changed inevitable in a pattern set down in its genetic material. This affects of matured behaviour was expected to occur in any kind of environment or socio-cultural context. Hall viewed the adolescence as the period of stress and storm. In his recapitulation theory, adolescence corresponds to the period when the human race was in turbulent and transitional stage. The following factors suggest that why people continue to believe in the storm and stress view of adolescence. First, many parents have their views that adolescence as a period of storm and stress because it is difficult for parents to let go their teenage child, and to give them independence. Hence, parents may become defensive in their reactions to the views of adolescence. Perhaps, as some have suggested, parents project the feelings of conflict and confusion they experience when their children become independent onto the adolescent, rather than them, and therefore, view the adolescence as the one who "is going through a period of storm and stress." Second, the media does much promote the storm and stress view of adolescence. The number of television programs give them a thought that deal with runways, juvenile gangs, drug addicts and teen-age prostitutes. It is no wonder that many are tempted to generalize from these specific instances to the adolescence population as a whole. Obviously, this is both unfair and unrealistic. Some theorists suggest that the interaction of biological and socio-cultural influences on development is independent strivings. The adolescence grows larger, more experienced, and more competent and knows it, and others must learn to adapt and react to these changes and the demands for independence the adolescent exerts, in part, because of these changes.

Cognitive-Development theories:

Jean Piaget developed a theory of cognitive-development that is fast becoming the most popular and perhaps most productive development theory in use today. Piaget (1952) proposed that intelligence develops in stages and reflects the emergence of biological predispositions as well as cultural influences. Piaget argues that from infancy through adulthood all humans function cognitively in the same trend. In other words, the way in which intelligence works is age-invariant. However, Piaget argues that there are stages of cognitive development that reflect qualitative differences in the structure of an individual's intelligence from infancy through adulthood. Structures, which are reflected in the individual's behavior, determine intellectual competencies. Since structures change with the age and with social interaction, competencies change, too. At adolescence the highest level of cognition, formal operational thinking, is reached. Early adolescence is characterized by concrete operational thinking, whereas later adolescence is characterized by formal operational thinking. In other words, the adolescent years span a change in cognitive development. Therefore, as adolescents become capable of formal operational thinking, their cognitive abilities as well as their views about external world change. In addition, adolescents are capable of not only asking, but also of coming up with some answers to such abstract questions as "who am I ?". Hence, it appears that Piaget's notions about cognitive development, which are based on a biological predisposition interacting with cultural demands, relate to certain aspects of adolescent behavior.

During the adolescent years, the individual is assumed to develop to the level of moral thinking that is dominant within the society. For now, it is sufficient to note that understanding of the social order may change developmentally and may achieve adult levels during the adolescent years. In part this is achieved through role taking (Selman, 1971), which is promoted by peer interaction. Role taking helps the adolescent to become capable of taking another's perspective. By examining the relationships between cognitive development and other behaviors, then, one can gain some insight into adolescent peer relations, personality development, and idealism in viewing sociopolitical systems. Indeed, it may well be that the changes in cognitive competence during adolescence are the keystones to understanding much of adolescent behavior.

Social Learning Theories:

Many researchers have noted, adolescence takes place within the confines of a society, a social structure. The nature of this social structure defines what is expected of adolescents and what avowable behavior is. Moreover, it is the social structure that defines the tasks of adolescence (Havighurst, 1972). In the other words, the society in which she/he grows up apparently has a significant impact on the adolescent. This point was brought home most directly and forcefully first by cultural anthropologists who have studied adolescents and, more recently, by social learning theorist, who espouse the importance of setting conditions, reinforces, and contexts in the study of development. Social learning theory, emphasize the role of the culture and the environment in explaining development. In addition, this theory also pays the attention to the importance of biological determinants of behavior. Social learning theorists believe that people form their thoughts, feelings, and actions from observing and intimate what they perceives to be the thoughts, feelings and actions of others.

Social learning theorists assume that adolescent behavior is simply the result of particular kinds of child rearing practices. The notion here is that a very few adolescents will exhibit deviant kinds of behaviors; most will exhibit behaviors that are relatively in harmony with the kinds of behaviors they were taught in childhood. This thinking simply reflects the notion of social learning theorists that, there is continuity in human growth patterns and learning processes and that at no particular age level should there be broad changes in behavior that might be due to what we call maturational development. Deviant development that emerges during the adolescent stage of life, then, is seen as a failure of socialization processes that were begun earlier in childhood. Children who are taught to behave adversely in stressful situations, which are taught to exhibit deviant behavior, or who did not learn to deal adequately with reality will, according to social learning theory view, exhibit similar kinds of behavior.

Therefore, social learning theories have described the impact of environment on development, but at a more fine-grained level. They would have explored of cultural factors in depth in order to comprehend adolescent development.

Psychodynamic theories-

The psychodynamic view of adolescence, or any other period of development, rests on several fundamental principles (Adelson & Doehrman, 1980). First, psychodynamic theories are historical in nature. That is, from this perspective one can understand the adolescent's current behavior only through reference to his or her past experiences and personal history. By knowing something of adolescent's development history, one can gain better understanding of current behavior, such as vocational choice. Second, psychodynamic theories are steeped in instinct theory. During adolescence, this emphasis has been translated into a focus on drives, such as the sex drive, that are viewed as increasing in strength. In this context the emphasis has been on the study on defense against the increase in drives. This perspective of adolescent development is well illustrated in the writings of Anna Freud (1948, 1958). Anna Freud, daughter of Sigmund Freud, attempted to spell out some of the dynamics of the psychoanalytic point of view (A. Freud, 1948) of adolescent development. Her view is that the behavior of adolescents is due to the sudden upsurges of sexuality which in turn, is due to the biological changes that occur during pubescence. Hence, maturational factors directly influence the psychological functioning. The increase in sexuality brings about a recurrence of the oedipal situation, which once again must be resolved. However, this time the resolution is through attraction to opposite sex peers. Because of the increase in to sexuality, the adolescent is viewed as being in the state of stress not very different from the stress created by the original oedipal situation. This stress produces anxiety, which, in turn, leads to the development of depression.

For many, adolescence is a time in life that coincides with many milestones of development (e.g., the onset of puberty or high school graduation). However, these celebratory events do not define the transition between childhood and adulthood. Throughout the literature, the term adolescence has been difficult to concretely define (Hine, 1999; Santrok, 2001). This may be due to the fact that adolescence requires consideration of multiple factors including age and contextual influences. In addition, adolescence is a cultural and social phenomenon causing difficulty in defining the beginning and endpoints of this development stage (Santrok, 2001). For example, within the Jewish community, adolescent males are considered an adult at the age of thirteen, and is directly associated with the Bar Mitzvah ceremony (a formal age of maturity). In contrast, many Western societies define adolescence within a much broader time period. For example, the United States recognizes adolescence between the ages of thirteen to twenty four years of age (Hine, 1999). The literature has suggested that adolescence is a relatively new phenomenon within Western societies and is viewed as a by-product of social pressures specific to culture (Hine, 1999). Compared to many other cultures, western societies have not defined adolescence as distinct phase of life. This causes uncertainty as to when adulthood begins, and how an individual makes the transition from childhood to adulthood.

Developmental Issues

Given that adolescence is a developmental period that constitutes potential for conflict as well as opportunities for growth, understanding the conflicts that arise for individuals attempting to overcome barriers and obstacles along their developmental path may provide insight into the development and expression of emotional difficulties. Numerous developmental theorists have attempted to explain the changes that occur in the period between childhood and adulthood. Many theories have been developed in an attempt to explain development in terms of stages, focusing on specific changes that occur at each stage, and progressing to the next stage in order to reach a functional level as an adult. For instance, Piaget's theory emphasized that a critical stage in adolescence was developing abstract thinking (Piaget, 1972). Another stage theorist, Eric Erikson (1968), focused on psycho-social stages within adolescent development proposing that this is a period where each adolescent formulates their own identity. The risk of identity confusion is included in Erikson's psychosocial stages identified as occurring in the transition between childhood and adulthood. Erikson (1968) describes this risk as feelings of isolation, doubt, anxiety and indecision. Furthermore, these traits may interfere with the individual's ability to enter the next stage of development.

Development has typically been described in the literature in terms of time periods. Three processes commonly determine adolescent development: biological, cognitive and socio-emotional (Santrok, 2001).

Biological processes consist of individuals' unique biological make-up that genetically influences behaviour and development. Biologically determined processes of development were dominant viewpoints in the early twentieth century. Stanley Hall often thought of as the father of scientific study of adolescence, applied the scientific and biological dimensions of Darwin's Theory of Evolution in the study of adolescence. Hall believed that development was predominantly biologically determined, and environmental factors played a minimal role. It is important to note that although he viewed development as predominantly biological, Hall did incorporate environmental accounts for change in development during adolescence (Hall, 1904). Current thought emphasizes the fact that biology does play a critical role in development, although theories are now attempting to identify how biological processes interact with environmental processes in adolescent development.

Cognitive processes incorporate that which changes in individual thinking throughout the course of development. This view emphasizes that adolescents have sophisticated thinking abilities and are motivated to understand and construct their owncognitive worlds. Theorists focus on individual differences involving complex cognitive abilities including problem solving abilities, memory capacity, decision making. Current strides within this perspective include examining how individuals within this age group apply critical thinking and are able to adapt competently within their environment.

Cognitive processes have implications for creating educational programs during the process of development. Socio-emotional processes involve the development of individual emotions in relation to social context and other people. Research suggests that important contexts in adolescent development include family, peer, school and cultural contexts. In addition to particular contexts in which individuals are encompassed, social and personality development (e.g., gender roles, identity, sexuality and achievement) interact with environmental situations to further complicate this process. Research in this field has focused on developmental and contextual factors involved in healthy or unhealthy development.

In summary, biological, cognitive and socio-emotional processes are intricately related and constantly interacting. Changes in adolescent development are an outcome of all processes involved.

ANXIETY, DEPRESSION AND ADOLOSCENTS

Depression and anxiety are the two most common reasons for adolescent referrals for treatment. It has become clear within the literature that depression and anxiety are major, pervasive, and debilitating aspects of adolescent development (Santrok, 2001).

Often referred to as the common cold of mental disorders, both anxiety and depression are debilitating conditions that greatly impair psychological, social and emotional well-being. Moreover, such consequences place significant strain on interpersonal relationships and present an economic cost to society (Dozois & Dobson, 2004; Barlow, 2002; Gotlib & Hammen, 2002). Given the fact that anxiety and depression tax the resources of both individuals and society, it is important for researchers to develop models to aid in understanding the development of these disorders; especially in terms of the relationship between sub-clinical anxiety and depression in normal populations. Understanding sub-clinical anxiety and depression can facilitate the development of early intervention strategies.

For millennia, humans have experienced and sought to understand anxiety and depression (e.g., Plato and Aristotle). Researchers continue to develop and test theory based constructs to explain the disorders. Anxiety and depression possess aspects that are both normative and debilitating to one's life. Sigmund Freud aptly summarized this viewpoint in the following words "One thing is certain, that the problem of anxiety is a nodal point, linking up all kinds of the most important questions; a riddle of which the solution must cast a flood of light upon our whole mental life" (Barlow & Durand, 2005, p. 250).

Several psychological theories have examined anxiety, depression and the relationship between both constructs. For example, psychodynamic, behavioural, cognitive and, more recently, integrated theories, have all attempted to explain the distinct and overlapping features of anxiety and depression.

Psychodynamic theories have focused mainly on underlying unresolved conflicts that individuals express through the symptomologies of anxiety and depression. Sigmund Freud viewed anxiety as a defence mechanism for repressed and unconscious impulses (Davison, Neale, Blankstein & Flett, 2005). Similarly, many psychoanalysts have pondered the point that depressed individuals harbour unconscious negative feelings towards those they love, causing anger to turn inward (Davison et al., 2005). Freud posited that this is a defence mechanism to cope with socially unacceptable feelings. Unfortunately, there is little empirical evidence to support these psychodynamic assumptions (Barlow & Durand, 2005; Davison, et al., 2005; Kandel, 1999).

Behavioural theorists view anxiety and depression as a product of learning, where learned behavioural patterns contribute to the development of symptoms through processes such as modeling and classical conditioning. Furthermore, anxiety has been linked to a sense of little to no control over perceived future events within the environment (Chorpita & Barlow, 1998). Similarly, stressful events are identified in the etiology of depression (Barlow & Durand, 2005). The behavioural model more or less assumes that psychopathology is environmentally determined.

Cognitive theorists posit that assessing unique cognitive content would enable clinicians and researchers to distinguish between anxiety and depression (Beck & Perkins, 2001). More specifically, depressive cognitive content would reflect related cognitions conceptualized in Beck's Negative Cognitive Triad consisting of negative assessment of self, the world and future (Beck, 1976). It was hypothesized that depression reflects a cognitive content that encompassed themes of negative selfevaluation, hopelessness and a general pessimistic assessment of the world (Clark, Beck & Stewart, 1990). By contrast, cognitive theorists have proposed that anxiety-based cognitive content is related to concerns of physical or psychological threat (Beck & Perkins, 2001). Yet, understanding anxiety and depression as unique constructs has been further clouded by the consistent finding of high correlations of scores on self-report scales assessing symptoms of depression and anxiety (Dobson, 1985).

Behavioural and cognitive theories of depression and anxiety empirically support and fundamentally inform clinical practice. Over time, behavioural and cognitive models for depression and anxiety have become more complex. For example, the hopelessness and negative cognitive triad models of depression have evolved into the stress-diathesis model of depression. Similarly, integrating numerous factors, Barlow (2000; 2002) has developed the triple vulnerability theory that includes anxiety and related disorders. This theory speculates that the development of anxiety and related disorders, most commonly depression, are a result of numerous vulnerabilities that interact with environmental stressors (Barlow, 2000; 2002). This interaction encompasses aspects of both biological contributions and psychological contributions that underlie individual vulnerability.

During the 1980s, cognitive theorists investigated the overlap of anxiety and depression partly in response to diagnostic and assessment issues regarding the relationship of each unique construct (Beck & Perkins, 2001). Diagnostically, anxiety and depression are two distinct constructs, both encompassing multiple forms. Recent findings, however, have demonstrated that anxiety and depression overlap. For example, Barlow (2002) stated that the genetics of anxiety and depression are closely related, as is the neurobiology and the nature of individual vulnerability to each. Barlow (2002) points out that a temporal relationship may exist in that some people with vulnerability react with anxiety to life stressors and others react further to become depressed. While conceptually distinct, anxiety and depression are psychological phenomena more likely to have a complex etiological relationship. The need to understand etiology highlights the importance of studying the relationship between sub-clinical anxiety and depression in normal populations.

In sum, a current theory involving anxiety and depression recognizes the importance of drawing attention to the overlap of symptoms. Examining the relationship between anxiety and depression and attempts to discriminate one syndrome from the other seem to be the current theoretical and clinical focus among researchers and clinicians.

In recent years, there has been an increase in empirical support and research in the domains of anxiety and depression. Models of anxiety and depression have been developed from different theoretical backgrounds. Furthermore, models of anxiety and depression have guided the development of effective treatments. For years, a controversy has existed between the nature and nurture debate as it relates to psychopathology. In recognition of the importance of the gene-environment interaction, the diatheses-stress model was developed to explain why individuals who inherit the tendency to express a specific trait or behaviour might not exhibit the behaviour unless an environment stressor triggers activation of the trait (Barlow & Durand, 2005).

In treatment, precise diagnosis is paramount when formulating appropriate care plans for individuals dealing with the crippling effects of anxiety and depression. Anxiety and depression describe distinct phenomena, at least theoretically: anxiety is based upon fear while depression is based upon loss (Rutter & Rutter, 1992). What then makes a person vulnerable to developing anxiety, depression, or both? An environmental stressor enters the diathesis to activate the expression of a particular trait or behaviour. Multiple paths to a given outcome of anxiety or depression must exist because not all individuals with an inherited vulnerability express or terminate a particular trait or behaviour, or encounter a threshold of environmental stressors. Complex interactions between psychological and biological factors may alter various stages of development leading to different pathways and developmental outcomes.

Researchers not only examine what makes people exhibit particular disorders, but also how those who are at risk or who are vulnerable might be protected (Barlow & Durand, 2005).

While a substantial effort has been invested in the treatment of acute phases of anxiety and depression, few studies examine risk and vulnerability factors, or factors that may prevent sub-clinical anxiety and depression from reaching clinical levels. There is a current need for research on models that conceptualize sub-clinical states of anxiety and depression. For example, epidemiological studies that have examined adolescent populations have focused mainly on the prevalence of anxiety and depressive disorders as defined by the Diagnostic and Statistical Manual of Mental Disorders (DSM-IV) or International Classification of Diseases (ICD) criteria. By placing emphasis on subclinical symptoms of anxiety and depression, researchers may begin to understand the etiology that underlies the development of anxiety and depression as opposed to normative development.

Depression is one of the leading causes of morbidity and mortality in the world today and places profound economic burden on society (Greenberg, Kessler, Birnbaum, 2003& Lynch, Clarke, 2006). Youth depression is quite common (Kovacs, 2006) and is associated with negative long-term psychiatric and functional outcomes(Bar done, Moffitt, 1996 & Weismann, Wok, Goldstein, 1999) such as including impairment in school, work, and interpersonal relationships, substance abuse and suicide attempts (Rubin, Both, Zahn-Waxler, 1991 andZahn-Waxler, Dodge, Valence, 1995).

The depression is the most prevalent mental illness in present century; it's considered as the most serious illness and as Harvard University reported, it will be in the top of prevalent illnesses list by 2020. It is a mental disorder that affects one's thinking, feelings, behaviors and physical performance (Butler, 2002, cite by Aston et al, 2004).

Depression incurs nearly 12% of world's population to pay heavy expenses (Aston et al, 2004). Normally the cost which incurs by a depressed person is much more than those incurred by victims of other illnesses (Vakili et al, 2009). Economists estimated that depression incurs 43 billion dollars to the U.S.A. per year (Hunter, 2009). According to DSM-IV, depression could be detected by 8 main features: bad mood (at least for two weeks), dissatisfaction in many activities, disorders while sleeping, significant changes in weight, lack of energy, emptiness or guilt, disorders in concentration, suicide thoughts and contemplations (Greenberg & Watson, 2007).

15% of depressed ills die of suicide. Studies show that 1,000,000 people die of suicide in the world per year; in other words, one per 30 seconds (Hunter, 2009).

Studies have proved that kids and teenagers suffer from depression as adults do and these disorders affect their performance and whole lives (Neshatdust, 2007). Teenagers pass the childhood towards adulthood; many of them experience personal and family problems during this period (Lindsey et al, 2000 cited by Kameli, 2009).

Anxiety disorders are the most frequent mental health problem in children and adolescents, with prevalence rates estimated to be around 10-15% /.Adolescence is an important time window in the development of anxiety disorders, as 75% of all cases of anxiety disorders have their onset between ages 11 and 21 years. Furthermore, many anxiety disorders in adolescents are characterized by low rates of remission if untreated .

School psychologists assist children and adolescents to succeed academically, socially, behaviorally, and emotionally (National Association of School Psychologist.). They are highly trained in psychology and education and aim to deliver comprehensive and integrated services. As indicated within the National Association of School Psychologists' (NASP) *Model for Comprehensive and Integrated School Psychological Services* (2010), school psychologists should aid in the development and implementation of interventions and mental health services to foster student development of social and life skills. With their knowledge of biological, cultural, developmental, and social influences on mental health, school psychologists are capable of providing a continuum of mental health services, including individual and group counseling (NASP, 2010). In a recent survey study sampling school psychologists across the United States, reporting school psychologists dedicate approximately 9% of their time to individual student group counseling and conducting student groups (Castillo, Curtis & Gelley, 2012).

School psychologists recognize that good mental health is important. As conceptualized by NASP, mental health is not simply the absence of mental illness; it also means having the skills necessary to cope with life's challenges (NASP, n.d.). Here, school psychologists can serve as mental health professionals and prevent or reduce the immediate and long-term consequences of mental health problems experienced by children. In addition, school psychologists can take leadership roles to support systems level services to address the mental health and welfare of all students and bring increased attention to the need for schools to address these areas to ensure effective academic development (Ysseldyke et al., 2006).

In a recent study that surveyed school psychologists, perceived knowledge, role preference, and training needs regarding the prevention and treatment of internalizing disorders, the majority of school psychologists indicated that prevention of internalizing disorders, including anxiety, is well within the role of a school psychologist (Miller & Jome, 2010). Moreover, depending on the nature of the disorder, school psychologists' opinions about treating disorders differed. There was a strong consensus that school psychologists should prevent and treat children with school refusal behaviors. In addition, half of the sample agreed that school psychologists should aid in the treatment of anxiety disorders.

Taking all the information together, anxiety disorders are common in youth. If left untreated, the disorders worsen over time and are associated with a host of negative outcomes. Therefore, early identification and treatment for anxious youth should be a priority. Recently, schools have become the primarily access point for mental health services. Schools are ideal venues for treatment delivery, because they overcome many of the traditional obstacles inherent in community or in private based treatments (i.e., cost, transportation, stigma, etc).

Furthermore, many randomized clinical trial studies have demonstrated the efficacy of CBT to treat anxiety disorders in children and are showing promising results for effectively treating children in schools. Also, behavioral consultation has shown to be effective for treating children with anxiety disorders. However, the one shortcoming is that most rely on a professional mental health clinician for treatment delivery.

Therefore, training and accessing school-based personnel for treatment delivery has received much attention. In the school setting, school psychologists are in an ideal position to identify and treat anxious and depressed youth. They have the training to support children with mental health needs. In addition, providing school-based treatments to student with mental health needs is within the role and scope of comprehensive services provided by school psychologists.

REVIEW OF LITERATURE

REVIEW OF LITERATURE

This review of literature focuses on the interventions for adolescents to work on optimism, rumination, anxiety and depression. These interventions need good counselors and psychology professionals to work. Thus this also includes some of the studies showing how it is important for any educational institute having adolescent population to have at least one psychology professional in their premises.

Anxiety and counseling

Study on Efficacy of Modular Cognitive Behavior Therapy for Childhood Anxiety Disorders by Bruce E. Chorpita et al. in 2013 evaluated the initial efficacy of a modular approach to cognitive behavior therapy (CBT) for anxiety disorders in youth. Modular CBT consists of the guided combination of individually scripted techniques that are explicitly matched to the child's individual strengths and needs. Eleven youth primarily of Asian and Pacific Island ethnicity ranging in age from 7 to 13 were referred for treatment. Comparisons in a multiple baseline across children provided preliminary support for the efficacy of the intervention. Among the 7 completers, all principal diagnoses were absent at post treatment and 6-month follow-up assessments, and measures of anxiety symptoms and life functioning almost uniformly evidenced clinically significant improvements.

A qualitative study on the implementation of the friends anxiety management and mental health promotion program by Kafui Abra Sawyer in 2011. This study was an exploration of what helps and hinders educators in their decisions regarding the implementation of the FRIENDS anxiety management as designed by the licensee. An environmental scan undertaken by the Ministry of Children and Family Development in Chilliwack, British Columbia, revealed that the program is delivered with limited attention to treatment fidelity and some schools choose not to implement. Semi-structured interviews were conducted with 12 educators using the critical incident technique. 773 incidents emerged from the interviews: 441 helpful, 263 hindering and 69 wish list items. Educators reported that their personal views about the value, importance and benefit of the FRIENDS program as well as the support received from school administrators proved helpful in decisions regarding implementation. Educators also indicated that time commitment and sense of competency hindered their training and implementation decisions. Implications for practice include the value of emphasizing self-efficacy dynamics and of providing influential persons as support networks when promoting school-based mental health programs. This research may offer heuristic value for policy makers, managers and program developers.

A pilot study utilizing cross-age peer tutoring as a method of intervention for anxious adolescents was done by Dr Marilyn Campbell (2008). The study was about anxiety disorders are the most common psychopathology experienced by young people, with up to 18% of adolescents developing one. The consequences of these symptoms, if left untreated, include impaired peer relationships, school absenteeism and self-concept problems. In addition, excessive anxiety may play a causal role in the development of depression in young people, precede eating disorders and predispose adolescents to substance abuse disorders. While the school is often chosen as a place to provide early intervention for these debilitating symptoms, identifying sufferers is difficult because excessive anxiety is often not recognized in school and young people are reluctant to seek help. Even when these young people are identified, there are problems in providing sensitive programs that do not stigmatize them within a school setting. One method that may engage this adolescent population is cross-age peer tutoring. They used Worry busters program and a cross-age peer tutoring method to engage anxious adolescents. Secondary school students with anxiety were invited to plan activities for primary school students who had been referred by a teacher as also suffering from anxiety. The secondary students prepared the activities across the course of a term in the high school setting, and then delivered them to the younger students in weekly sessions at the primary school during the following term. Although the secondary school students decreased their scores on anxiety self-report measures, there were no significant differences in primary school students' self-reports.

Psychosocial interventions to prevent anxiety disorders in school settings from 1985–2007: a meta-analysis done by Julia Gallegos, Raquel Benavides, Tasha Beretvas and Sylvia Linan-Thompson. Their study revealed that Childhood anxiety disorders are a salient concern because they are associated with deviant conduct, substance abuse, and depression later in life. This meta-analysis focuses on the efficacy of psychosocial interventions in preventing anxiety disorders in children. A search of several databases covering 1985- 2007 identified 19 peer-reviewed studies. Most of the studies were judged with "Low Risk of Bias". Results showed CBT to be the most effective psychosocial intervention (95% CI, 0.19 a 0.43), particularly when implemented at a selective prevention level (95% CI, 0.20 a 0.97). The protective factors to improve the most were positive future outlook (95% CI, 0.87 to 1.51) and self-esteem (95% CI, 0.87 a 1.51).

Larun, Nordheim, Ekeland, Hagen and Heian (2006) assessed the effect of exercise interventions in reducing or preventing anxiety or depression in children and young people up to 20 years of age. The trials were combined using meta-analysis method. Results show that the depression scores showed a statistically significant difference in favor of the exercise group. They conclude that there appears to be an effect in favor of exercise in reducing depression and anxiety scores in the general population of children and adolescents.

Lee and Overholser (2006) developed an integrated treatment plan for person with depression and personality dysfunction. The challenges encountered by the therapist include: (i) differentiating borderline personality from depressive symptoms. (ii) maintaining the therapeutic alliance (iii) managing impulsivity and self-destructive tendencies (iv) staying focused on long term therapeutic goals and (v) coping with non compliance. Over the course of 27 sessions, the client was able to make positive changes in mood, self-image and impulsive tendencies. Although the client's border line personality traits complicated the course of treatment for depression, neglecting these personality problems would have left the client vulnerable to depressive relapse.

Another study titled as Prevention and intervention for anxiety disorders in children and adolescents: A whole school approach done by Marilyn A Campbell in 2003. This study explores a whole school approach to the prevention and intervention for anxiety disorders in children and adolescents. Anxiety disorders are the most prevalent psychopathology in childhood and adolescence. In addition to having serious consequences for academic, social and family life, anxiety has also been shown to be a precursor to depression, substance abuse and eating disorders. School counselors are well placed to identify students with anxiety disorders, instigate prevention programs and reat or refer anxious students. Prevention and early intervention for anxiety disorders needs to be co-ordinate and integrated into the regular curriculum as well as into the life of the classroom and the school. Barriers to schools working well in this area are identified and discussed.

A community-based nursing study was conducted by Sloman (2002) in Sydney, Australia to compare the effects of progressive muscle relaxation and guided imagery on anxiety and quality of life in people with advanced cancer. In the study, 56 people with advanced Cancer who were experiencing anxiety and depression were randomly assigned to 1 of 4 treatment conditions: (1) Progressive muscle relaxation training, (2) guided imagery training, (3)both of these treatment and (4) control group. Subjects were tested before and after learning muscle relaxation and guided imagery technique for anxiety, depression and quality of life using the Hospital Anxiety and Depression Scale and the Functional Living Index Cancer Scale. Results show that there is no significant improvement for anxiety; however, significant positive changes occurred for depression and quality of life.

Depression, anxiety and optimism

A. Man Yee Ho et al. found the role of meaning in life and optimism in 2010. This study examined the relationship between meaning in life, optimism and well-being among adolescents. A total of 1807 adolescents in Hong Kong completed inventories that assessed their personality, psychosocial problems and life satisfaction. Results of structural equation modeling (SEM) indicated that both meaning in life and optimism significantly associated with multidimensional life satisfaction and multidimensional structure of psychosocial problems among adolescents. Optimism also served as a partial mediator in the relationships between meaning in life and both positive and negative aspects of well-being. The mediating role of optimism did not differ across gender.

Liza Day & John Maltby found the role of optimism in irrational belief in 2010. The authors examined the relationship of belief in good luck with depression and anxiety within the context of a number of cognitive and personality variables used to explain depression and anxiety. Undergraduate students (46 men, 98 women) were administered measures of belief in good luck, depression, anxiety, optimism, neuroticism, attribution style, self-esteem, and irrational beliefs. The results showed that belief in good luck was significantly related to optimism and irrational beliefs. A number of models were tested to determine whether irrational beliefs or optimism mediated the relationship between belief in good luck and depression and anxiety. The findings suggested that negative relationships between belief in good luck and both depression and anxiety are best addressed by the theory that belief in good luck engenders optimistic traits and a reduced level of irrational beliefs.

Hope vs optimism as Contributions to depression and life satisfaction by Shyh ShinWong and Timothy Lim in 2009. This study explored the discriminant validity of optimism and hope in accounting for unique variance in depression and life satisfaction for 334 secondary school students from Singapore. Correlational analysis showed that optimism and hope were significantly correlated with each other. Hierarchical multiple regression findings indicated that both optimism and hope significantly predicted depression and life satisfaction even after controlling for hope and optimism, respectively. However, the incremental unique variance accounted for in depression by optimism is 6% more than that accounted for by hope in terms of R^2 *Change* values. Simultaneous multiple regression analyses using the subscale scores found that only agency, optimism, and pessimism contributed uniquely to the variance in depression and life satisfaction. Implications and limitations of these findings are discussed.

A longitudinal study of the effects of pessimism, trait anxiety, and life stress on depressive symptoms in middle-aged women was done by Bromberger, Joyce T.; Matthews, Karen A. in 1996. The relative contributions of life stress, menopausal status, and pessimism and trait anxiety during the presence and absence of stress on increases in depressive symptoms across 3 years were examined in a sample of 460 premenopausal women, aged 42-50, who had few depressive symptoms at study entry. Multivariate analyses showed that after statistical adjustments for initial depressive symptoms and education, depressive symptoms at follow-up were higher among women (a) who reported stressful events, especially of a chronic nature, (b) who scored highly on trait anxiety, and (c) who were pessimistic and subsequently experienced a stressful ongoing problem. Change in menopausal status was not related to symptoms. The study confirms that midlife stress and both optimism and trait anxiety are important predictors of depressive symptoms during midlife.

The specificity of attribution style and expectations to positive and negative affectivity, depression, and anxiety by Ahrens, A.H. and Haaga (1993). Ninety-four undergraduate subjects completed measures of trait positive and negative affectivity, anxiety, depression, optimism, hopelessness, and attributional style. Attributional style predicted state positive affect following completion of negative essays, but not negative affect, nor either affect following the positive tape. Effects of attributional style on affect were partially independent of expectations. Results are discussed in terms of the importance of distinguishing between processes related to positive and negative affect in order to distinguish anxiety from depression.

Michael B. Frisch did a study on Quality of Life Therapy and Coaching (also known as Quality of Life Therapy) in 2013. This study was a comprehensive, manualized, theory-based, and, according to Diener (2013) and Seligman (Flourish, Free Press, NY, 2011, p. 292), evidence-based approach to well being, happiness, and positive psychology intervention suitable for both coaching and clinical applications. Clients are taught strategies and skills aimed at helping them to identify, pursue, and fulfill their most cherished needs, goals, and wishes in sixteen valued areas of life said to comprise human well-being and happiness. Quality of Life Therapy and Coaching is "manualized" in the form of the book entitled Quality of Life Therapy (Frisch 2006), providing step-by-step instruction in assessing well-being, tailoring interventions, and monitoring progress, outcome, and follow-up with the evidence-based well-being assessment, the Quality of Life Inventory or QOLL. This article describes Quality of Life Therapy and Coaching and reviews developments and research since the publication of the manual in 2006. Randomized controlled trials bearing on the empirical support of Quality of Life Therapy and Coaching and the related assessment, the Quality of Life Inventory, are reviewed. The steps in Quality of Life Therapy and Coaching are delineated in the context of an illustrative case and an underlying theory which attempts to integrate findings from the fields of well-being, positive psychology, happiness, quality of life, social indicators research, psychotherapy, and coaching.

Depression and counseling

Depression interventions for adolescents most commonly take the approach of cognitive-behavioral group therapy. The basic premise of cognitive-behavioral therapy is that our thoughts impact our emotions, which in turn impact our behavior. Cognitive-behavioral approaches typically teach cognitive restructuring skills, which assist participants in identifying and challenging their negative, unconstructive thoughts.

Depression is one of the leading causes of morbidity and mortality in the world today and places profound economic burden on society (Greenberg, Kessler, Birnbaum, 2003& Lynch, Clarke, 2006). Youth depression is quite common (Kovacs, 2006) and is associated with negative long-term psychiatric and functional outcomes (Bar done, Moffitt, 1996 & Weismann, Wok, Goldstein, 1999) such as including impairment in school, work, and interpersonal relationships, substance abuse and suicide attempts (Rubin, Both, Zahn-Waxler, 1991 and Zahn-Waxler, Dodge, Valence, 1995). The depression is the most prevalent mental illness in present century; it's considered as the most serious illness and as Harvard University reported, it will be in the top of prevalent illnesses list by 2020.

It is a mental disorder that affects one's thinking, feelings, behaviors and physical performance (Butler, 2002, cite by Aston et al, 2004). Depression incurs nearly 12% of world's population to pay heavy expenses (Aston et al, 2004). Normally the cost which incurs by a depressed person is much more than those incurred by victims of other illnesses (Vakili et al, 2009). Economists estimated that depression incurs 43 billion dollars to the U.S.A. per year (Hunter, 2009).

According to DSM-IV, depression could be detected by 8 main features: bad mood (at least for two weeks), dissatisfaction in many activities, disorders while sleeping, significant changes in weight, lack of energy, emptiness or guilt, disorders in concentration, suicide thoughts and contemplations (Greenberg & Watson, 2007). 15% of depressed ills die of suicide. Studies show that 1,000,000 people die of suicide in the world per year; in other words, one per 30 seconds (Hunter, 2009). Studies have proved that kids and teenagers suffer from depression as adults do and these disorders affect their performance and whole lives (Neshatdust, 2007).

A meta-analysis of school-based depression prevention programs for children and adolescents was done by Sherry L. Cowen 2014. School-based depression prevention programs are being implemented in schools across the world in efforts to inoculate children and adolescents from depressive symptoms. This met analysis examined 56 manuscripts with a total of 82 studies which focused on school-based programs to determine how they affect depression, anxiety, cognitive skills, self-esteem, coping, and internalizing behaviors. For these specific outcomes, effect sizes ranged from .08 to .25. All combined outcomes yielded a significant effect size of .15. Moderator analyses revealed key differences that identified characteristics of the most effective programs. Targeted programs servicing at-risk students yielded an effect size of .31, while universal programs produced a significant but small effect size of .07. However, the program facilitator seemed to impact the effectiveness of all types of programs.

Non-school personnel produced a .39 effect size with targeted samples, and .17 with universal samples, while school personnel produced about one half to a third of the effect.

The study of solution-focused group counseling in decreasing depression among teenage girls was the study conducted by Leila Javanmiri, Seyyed Ali Kimiaee, Bahram Ali Ghanbari and Hashem Abadi in 2012. The aim of this study is to determine the effect of solution-focused approach in decreasing depression among teenage girls. Depression is one of the most common diseases in these days which have been known as mental flu. Adolescence also plays a pivotal and key role in our in which depression is very common. So it is necessary to treat this disorder in adolescence. This research was a quasi-experimental design in which pretest-posttest design with a control group has been used. The population was all teenage girls in Sahneh; 20 girls were drawn from the population through stratified random sampling and then randomly assigned to two groups: one experimental and one control. Data were collected through Beck's depression questionnaire (BDI). Dependent variable was solution-focused therapy in which experimental group was provided with 8-hour group counseling (8 sessions which took one hour). In the meantime, control group was provided with irrelevant teachings (teaching study skills) to eliminate the effect of subjects. After the sessions were wound up, BDI questionnaire was administered again among both groups. One month later, the posttest and then BDI questionnaire were conducted. After that, t test and covariance were used to analyze the findings. The results showed that solution-focused group counseling is effective in decreasing depression among teenage girls and its significance level is at $\alpha= 0/01$. In addition, the findings obtained through posttest indicated how stable the effect of therapy is. In other words, solution-focused group counseling has significantly led to decreasing depression in teenage girls.

Other common elements of cognitive behavioral group therapy include "the focus on specific and current actions and cognitions as targets for change, structured intervention sessions, repeated practice of skills, use of rewards and contracts, homework assignments, and a relatively small (typically under 20) number of therapy sessions" (Rhode et al., 2005, p. 221).

A Brief Behavioral Activation Treatment for Depression C. W. Lejuez Derek R. Hopko And Sandra D. Hopko (2003).The brief behavioral activation treatment for depression (BATD) is a relatively uncomplicated, time-efficient, and cost-effective method for treating depression. Because of these features, BATD may represent a practical intervention within managed care–driven, inpatient psychiatric hospitals. Based on basic behavioral theory and empirical evidence supporting activation strategies, we designed a treatment to increase systematically exposure to positive activities and thereby help to alleviate depressive affect. This study represents a pilot study that extends research on this treatment into the context of an inpatient psychiatric unit. Results demonstrate effectiveness and superiority of BATD as compared with the standard supportive treatment provided within the hospital. A large effect size was demonstrated, despite a limited sample size.

Richard O'Kearney et al. 2008 did a school-based Internet program for reducing depressive symptoms in adolescent girls. This study evaluates the benefits of a self-directed Internet intervention for depression) delivered as a part of the high school curriculum. One hundred and fifty-seven girls, aged 15 and 16 years, were allocated to undertake either or their usual curriculum. Intervention impact on depressive symptoms, risk of depression, attributional style, depression literacy and attitudes toward depression was examined using random effect regression. Intervention produced a significantly faster rate of decline in depressive symptoms over the trial period than the control condition. The effect size for intervention was not significant immediately after the intervention (Cohen's d=.19, 95% CI −.18–.56) but was moderate and significant 20 weeks after the intervention (d=.46, 95% CI .10–.82). Girls with high depression scores before intervention showed the strongest benefits on self-reported depression at follow-up (d=.92, 95% CI .10–1.38). There were no significant intervention effects on depression status, attribution style, depression literacy, and attitudes. Approximately 70% of girls in the intervention group completed less than three of its modules and completion of fewer modules was related to high depression score before intervention. The findings suggest that there are benefits from intervention on self-reported depressive symptoms but has low rates of completion highlight problems in ensuring adherence to Internet programs for depression.

A study by Bolton and Bass (2007) investigated the objective of assessing the effect of locally feasible interventions on depression and anxiety among adolescent survivors of war and displacement in Northern Uganda. The intervention methods are locally developed screening tools that assessed the effectiveness of interventions in reducing symptoms of depression and anxiety. Activity based intervention (creative play) Interpersonal Psychotherapy was used with individuals wait listed to receive treatment at study end. The measure is a decrease in score on a depression symptom scale.

In the study Ellias and Bernard (2006) examined the effectiveness of cognitive behavioural therapy to childhood disorders. They found that individuals who can accept events and attributes no matter how negative, will experience natural feelings of disappointment and frustration, but will rarely manifest clinical depression. The increasing prevalence of depression in the child and adolescent population practitioners would be well advised to consider this approach in the prevention and treatment of depression in young clients. To promote school-based prevention programs that teach the connection between thoughts, feelings and behaviours, combined with a comprehensive intervention approach will hopefully empower young people to deal with this serious mental health problem.

A study reports on the efficacy of Cognitive Behavioral Therapy (CBT), Adolescent Skill Training - a group indicated preventive intervention (Young, Mufson and Davies, 2006). Adolescents in the two intervention conditions are compared on depression symptoms. The results show that adolescents who receive Cognitive Behavioral Therapy and Adolescent Skill Training have significantly fewer depression symptoms and better overall functioning at post-intervention and at follow-up.

Aniljose and Asha (2002) examined the efficiency of creativity training among children at risk of depression. Subject's were divided into two groups experimental and control groups. Experimental groups were given one month creativity training as a package. The results show that creativity training is effective for children at risk of depression and experimental group shows more symptom reduction than control group.

Marcotte (1996) examined the efficacy of cognitive behavioural therapy on adolescent depression. Results suggest that short-term group cognitive behavioural interventions are effective with early and late adolescents. Treatment components included relaxation, cognitive restructuring, self-control skills, communication and problem solving skills.

No single strategy seems to be more effective than the other.

In a study Janowick and Hackman (1995) explored the efficacy of assertiveness training and relaxation in promoting self-esteem and changes in depressive symptoms among adolescents. Two groups were given assertiveness training and a yogic relaxation technique referred to as *shavasana*. Pre and post test measures were taken on the personal orientation inventory and behavioural relaxation scale. Both groups showed significant increases in scores on self esteem and decreased scores on depression.

Alexander (1995) reviewed literature comparing relaxation and meditation techniques. Meta-analysis shows transcendental meditation (TM) to be significantly more effective than other forms of relaxation or meditation in (i) reducing psycho-physiological arousal (ii) reducing stress (iii) increasing positive mental health on measures of self esteem and (iv) reducing alcohol, nicotine, and illicit drug use relative to standard treatment and prevention programmes. Randomized controlled traits show that the TM technique significantly reduced hypertension and mortality in the elderly compared with a mental or physical relaxation technique.

In a study Chan (1993) examined the components of assertiveness and depressive symptoms of 183 Chinese University undergraduate students with their responses to Rathus Assertiveness Schedule and the Beck Depression Inventory. Three dimensions of assertiveness emerged: expressing, controlling and demanding responses. These components were found to relate differently to the beliefs in specific assertive rights, although there was no evidence that nonassertive behaviors could arise from beliefs that one did not have the rights to act assertively. Nonassertive responses, especially in expressing and disclosing oneself, correlated with depressed mood.

In an investigation by Burns and Hocksema (1991) factor analysis of the self-help inventory in a group of 307 consecutive outpatients seeking Cognitive Behavioural Therapy (CBT) for affective disorders revealed 3 factors that assessed the frequency with which subjects used active coping strategies when depressed, the perceived helpfulness of these coping strategies and their willingness to learn new coping strategies. The frequency and helpfulness scale do not predict patient's subsequent compliance with self-help assignments or their rate of improvement during the first 12 weeks of treatment. These findings suggest that very resourceful patients are not better candidates for CBT than other patients and that patients' expectations about the value of active coping strategies do not predict the response to CBT. In contrast the willingness scale was correlated with the degree of improvement during the first 12 weeks of treatment. The willingness scale and compliance with self help assignment made addictive separate contributions to clinical improvement.

Beck (1967, 1976), Beck and Young (1985), Young, Beck and Weinberger (1993) examined the role of deep-seated negative thinking in generating depression. The results show that negative thinking seems natural to them. Clients are taught that errors in thinking can directly cause depression. Treatment involves correcting cognitive errors and substituting less depressing and more realistic thoughts and appraisals. Sanchoz, Lewinsohn and Larson (1980), assigned depressed out patients (N= 32) to either group assertion training or 'traditional' group psychotherapy. The results show that over a relatively short period of time, assertiveness training is more effective than traditional Psychotherapy in increasing self-reported assertiveness and alleviating depression. In a study conducted by Hayman and Cope (1980) twenty-six moderately depressed females (mean age 21.3 yrs) were assigned randomly to assertiveness training. Results supported the effectiveness of treatment. Experimental subjects became significantly more assertive and engaged in significantly more activities than control subjects. Eight weeks after treatment, the experimental subjects' scores indicated significantly less depression. Other findings include significant negative correlations between measures of depression and assertiveness.

The study by Borkovec and Andrews (1987) examined thirty volunteers who met depressive symptoms and who received 12 sessions of training in progressive muscular relaxation. Sixteen of them were given cognitive therapy during 10 of those sessions and the remaining 14 received non directive therapy. Therapy was provided by 16 graduate student clinicians. The group as a whole showed substantial reductions in depressive symptoms and daily self-monitoring, although relaxation plus cognitive therapy produced significantly greater improvement than relaxation plus nondirective therapy. On several pre-therapy, post-therapy comparisons. Relaxation reduces depression and the results show significant positive relation between relaxation and outcomes.

Depression, Anxiety and Rumination

Rumination has captured the attention of researchers, including those studying emotion, social, clinical, developmental, and cognitive psychology (Papageorgiou & Wells, 2004; Wyer, 1996). Rumination has been defined as the tendency to focus repetitively on symptoms of emotional distress as well as the potential meaning, causes, and consequences of these symptoms without trying to solve the problems contributing to the emotional distress (Nolen-Hoeksema, 1991). Since Nolen-Hoeksema originally proposed Response Styles Theory (RST) and the concept of rumination, a large corpus of experimental, cross-sectional, and longitudinal studies, mostly among adults, has been conducted (see Lyubomirsky & Tkach, 2004; Thomson, 2006, for reviews). In addition, a handful of more recent studies have examined the association between rumination and depressive symptoms among children and adolescents Prospective studies of youth show that those who engage in ruminative responses to depressed mood are more likely to exhibit future elevations of depressive symptoms (e.g., Abela, Brozina, & Haigh, 2002; Abela, Vanderbilt, & Rochon, 2004; Broderick & Korteland, 2004; Burwell & Shirk, 2007; Nolen-Hoeksema, Stice, Wade & Bohon, 2007; Schwartz & Koenig, 1996; Ziegert & Kistner, 2002).

Targeting Ruminative Thinking in Adolescents at Risk for Depressive Relapse: Rumination Focused Cognitive Behavior Therapy in a Pilot Randomized Controlled Trial with Resting State in 2016 was done by Rachel H. Jacobs et.al. This pilot randomized control trial was designed to examine whether Rumination-Focused Cognitive Behavior Therapy (RFCBT) reduces rumination and residual depressive symptoms among adolescents with a history of Major Depressive Disorder (MDD) who are at risk for relapse. They also examined whether these changes in symptoms were associated with changes in functional connectivity of the posterior cingulated cortex (PCC), a key node in the default mode network (DMN). Thirty-three adolescents (ages 12–18) were randomized to eight weeks of RFCBT or an assessment only (AO) control. Twenty two adolescents successfully completed fMRI scans pre- and post-intervention. Adolescents were recruited from the clinic and community and met criteria for at least one previous episode of MDD and were currently in full or partial remission. Youth who received RFCBT also demonstrated significant decreases in connectivity between the left PCC and the right inferior frontal gyrus (IFG) and bilateral inferior temporal gyri (ITG). Degree of change in connectivity was correlated with changes in self-report depression and rumination. These data suggest that rumination can be reduced over eight weeks and that this reduction is associated with parallel decreases in residual depressive symptoms and decreased functional connectivity of the left PCC with cognitive control nodes. These changes may enhance the ability of vulnerable youth to stay well during the transition to adulthood.

Jeremy Oliver, Patrick Smith, and Eleanor Leigh found rumination in young people with depression in 2015. They examined how young people with depression experience rumination. Seven young people with depression were interviewed about the cognitive content of their rumination episodes, the associated feelings, and any behavioural start and stop triggers. Interview transcripts were analysed using Interpretative Phenomenological Analysis (IPA). Participants reported experiencing rumination as a disorientating cognitive battle, in which they felt under attack. The process elicited sadness predominantly, but also anger and anxiety, with mood and rumination often maintaining each other. Interpersonal interaction played a key role in starting and stopping rumination episodes. CBT-based interventions specifically targeting the ruminative process may be important for young people with depression, particularly interventions which consider the impact of family members or other systemic factors on rumination behavior.

David A. Kalmbach, Vivek Pillai and Jeffrey A. Ciesla found correspondence of changes in depressive rumination and worry in women in 2015. In the study of 67 women, weekly ratings of general distress, anxious arousal, anhedonic depression, worry, and rumination were collected over 5 weeks. Analyses revealed that both rumination and worry were independently related to concurrent general distress (shared feature of depression and anxiety), but not anxious arousal or anhedonia (unique symptoms). Further, a positive feedback loop was observed involving depressive rumination — and its brooding component—predicting greater general distress the following week, and vice versa. These findings indicate that depressive rumination and worry do not distinguish between depression and anxiety disorders, and that both forms of negative repetitive thoughts are related to shared features of depression and anxiety. However, given the cyclical relationship between rumination and distress symptoms, rumination may be a more corrosive cognitive process in women.

Rumination as a mechanism linking stressful life events to symptoms of depression and anxiety: Longitudinal evidence in early adolescents and adults was done by Michl, Louisa C. et al. in 2013. In the current study, they examined whether social environmental experiences were associated with rumination. Specifically, they evaluated whether self-reported exposure to stressful life events predicted subsequent increases in rumination. They also investigated whether rumination served as a mechanism underlying the longitudinal association between self-reported stressful life events and internalizing symptoms. Self-reported stressful life events, rumination, and symptoms of depression and anxiety were assessed in 2 separate longitudinal samples. A sample of early adolescents (N = 1,065) was assessed at 3 time points spanning 7 months. A sample of adults (N = 1,132) was assessed at 2 time points spanning 12 months. In both samples, self-reported exposure to stressful life events was associated longitudinally with increased engagement in rumination. In addition, rumination mediated the longitudinal relationship between self-reported stressors and symptoms of anxiety in both samples and the relationship between self-reported life events and symptoms of depression in the adult sample. Identifying the psychological and neurobiological mechanisms that explain a greater propensity for rumination following stressors remains an important goal for future research. This study provides novel evidence for the role of stressful life events in shaping characteristic responses to distress, specifically engagement in rumination, highlighting potentially useful targets for interventions aimed at preventing the onset of depression and anxiety.

Anson Whitmer and Ian H. Gotlib (2011) conducted factor analyses on scores on the RRS scale from samples. They found support for the distinction between reflections and brooding in never depressed and formerly depressed individuals; they did not obtain this distinct factor structure in the currently depressed sample. They did, however, find evidence of a second factor in the depressed sample that we labeled 'intentional rumination.' The results of this study also suggested that an item from the reflection factor should be replaced with another item from the RRS scale. These findings indicate that the distinction between brooding and reflection is blurred in currently depressed individuals.

Amy H. Mezulis, Heather A. Priess and Janet Shibley Hyde in 2010 examined prospective associations between negative emotionality, rumination, and depressive symptoms in a community sample of 301 youth (158 female) followed longitudinally from birth to adolescence. Mothers reported on youths' negative emotionality (NE) at age 1, and youth self-reported rumination at age 13 and depressive symptoms at ages 13 and 15. Linear regression analyses indicated that greater NE in infancy was associated with more depressive symptoms at age 15, even after controlling for child gender and depressive symptoms at age 13. Moreover, analyses indicated that rumination significantly mediated the association between infancy NE and age 15 depressive symptoms in the full sample. When analyzed separately by gender, however, rumination mediated the relationship between NE and depressive symptoms for girls but not for boys. The results confirm and extend previous findings on the association between affective and cognitive vulnerability factors in predicting depressive symptoms and the gender difference in depression in adolescence, and suggest that clinical interventions designed to reduce negative emotionality may be useful supplements to traditional cognitive interventions for reducing cognitive vulnerability to depression.

Jeffrey Roelofs et al. in 2009 sought to test predictions of the response styles theory in a sample of children and adolescents. More specifically, a ratio approach to response styles was utilized to examine the effects on residual change scores in depression and anxiety. Participants completed a battery of questionnaires including measures of rumination, distraction, depression, and anxiety at baseline (Time 1) and 8–10 weeks follow-up (Time 2). Results showed that the ratio score of rumination and distraction was significantly associated with depressed and anxious symptoms over time. More specifically, individuals who have a greater tendency to ruminate compared to distracting themselves have increases in depression and anxiety scores over time, whereas those who have a greater tendency to engage in distraction compared to rumination have decreases in depression and anxiety symptoms over time. These findings indicate that a ratio approach can be used to examine the relation between response styles and symptoms of depression and anxiety in non-clinical children and adolescents.

Filip Raes in 2009 found Rumination and worry as mediators of the relationship between self-compassion and depression and anxiety .The mediating effects of rumination (with brooding and reflection components) and worry were examined in the relation between self-compassion and depression and anxiety. Two hundred and seventy-one nonclinical undergraduates completed measures of self-compassion, rumination, worry, depression and anxiety. Results showed that for the relation between self-compassion and depression, only brooding (rumination) emerged as a significant mediator. For anxiety, both brooding and worrying emerged as significant mediators, but the mediating effect of worry was significantly greater than that of brooding. The present results suggest that one way via which self-compassion has buffering effects on depression and anxiety is through its positive effects on unproductive repetitive thinking.

In a research article titled Rethinking Rumination (2008) Susan Nolen-Hoeksema, Blair E. Wisco and Sonja Lyubomirsky. The response styles theory (Nolen-Hoeksema, 1991) was proposed to explain the insidious relationship between rumination and depression. We review the aspects of the response styles theory that have been well-supported, including evidence that rumination exacerbates depression, enhances negative thinking, impairs problem solving, interferes with instrumental behavior, and erodes social support. Next, we address contradictory and new findings. Specifically, rumination appears to more consistently predict the onset of depression rather than the duration, but rumination interacts with negative cognitive styles to predict the duration of depressive symptoms. Contrary to original predictions, the use of positive distractions has not consistently been correlated with lower levels of depressive symptoms in correlation studies, although dozens of experimental studies show positive distractions relieve depressed mood. Further, evidence now suggests that rumination is associated with psychopathologies in addition to depression, including anxiety, binge eating, binge drinking, and self-harm. We discuss the relationships between rumination and worry and between rumination and other coping or emotion-regulation strategies. Finally, we highlight recent research on the distinction between rumination and more adaptive forms of self-reflection, on basic cognitive deficits or biases in rumination, on its neural and genetic correlates, and on possible interventions to combat rumination.

In 2008 Benjamin L. Hankin did a study on Rumination and Depression in Adolescence: Investigating Symptom Specificity in a Multiwave Prospective Study. This prospective, multiwave study investigated whether baseline rumination predicted prospective elevations in depressive symptoms specifically. Rumination was assessed at baseline in a sample of early and middle adolescents ($N = 350$, 6–10th graders). Symptom measures of depression, anxious arousal, general internalizing, and conduct/externalizing problems with good discriminant validity were assessed at four time points over a 5-month period. Results using hierarchical linear modeling show that rumination predicted prospective fluctuations in symptoms of depression and general internalizing problems specifically but not anxious arousal or externalizing problems. Rumination predicted increasing prospective trajectories of general internalizing symptoms. Baseline rumination interacted with prospective co-occurring fluctuations of anxious arousal and externalizing behaviors over time to predict the highest levels of prospective depressive symptoms. Rumination partly mediated the sex difference (girls > boys) in depressive and internalizing symptoms.

In 2007 Pablo Fernandez-Berrocal, Rocio Alcaide, and Natalio Extremera examined the relationship between emotional intelligence, anxiety and depression among adolescents. Two hundred and fifty high-school students were administered the Trait Meta-Mood Scale (TMMS), a self-report measure of emotional intelligence, along with measures of thought suppression, self-esteem, anxiety, and depression. It was hypothesized that emotional abilities would predict psychological adjustment above and beyond factors that have been previously associated with poor adjustment (i.e., selfesteem and thought suppression). The study revealed two main findings. First, self-reported ability to regulate mood (Emotional Repair) was positively related to self-esteem. Second, self-reported emotional intelligence was negatively related to levels of depression and anxiety. Specifically, the ability to discriminate clearly among feelings (Emotional Clarity) and the ability to selfregulate emotional states were associated with better psychological adjustment, independent of the effects of self-esteem and thought suppression.

Reflection, Depressive Symptoms, and Subtypes of Rumination in Adolescence: Associations between Brooding, Coping was title of the research done by Rebecca A. Burwell & Stephen R. Shirk in 2007. This study examined associations between rumination and depressive symptoms in early adolescence. Using a short-term longitudinal design, we evaluated relations between subtypes of rumination and both depressive symptoms and coping among a community sample of 168 adolescents (70 boys, 98 girls, age M = 13.58). Results provided support for brooding and self-reflective subtypes of rumination. Brooding, but not reflection, predicted the development of depressive symptoms over time, particularly for girls. Brooding was related to maladaptive disengagement coping strategies, whereas reflection was related to adaptive primary and secondary coping strategies. These results suggest that not all types of self-focus on emotion contribute to the maintenance or intensification of depressive symptoms.

R.J. Park, I.M. Goodyer and J.D. Teasdale did a study in 2004. Their study investigated the effects of induced rumination as compared to distraction on mood and categorical over general memory in adolescents with first episode Major Depressive Disorder (MDD), and the specificity of any effects to MDD. Three subject groups; adolescents with first episode MDD ($N = 75$), non-depressed psychiatric participants ($N = 26$) and community controls ($N = 33$) were recruited. An experimental design was used, with repeated measures of 'in the moment' depressed mood and categorical over general memory before and after rumination and distraction, induced on separate occasions and counterbalanced in order across participants. Results showed that in adolescents with MDD, induced rumination as compared to distraction differentially increased depressed mood. There were no significant differences in this effect between full current MDD participants and those in partial remission. This differential effect was also seen in community controls but was absent in non-MDD psychiatric participants. In addition, rumination as compared to distraction increased over general memories to negative cues in MDD participants, but this increase was not significantly related to mood change, and was specific to MDD, being absent in non-MDD psychiatric and community control groups. Experimentally induced rumination as compared to distraction increases depressed mood and negative categoric memories in adolescents with first episode MDD. These results suggest that rumination has a deleterious effect on mood and memory retrieval processes in adolescents with first episode MDD. Increased negative over general memories with rumination may be a process of particular importance for adolescents with MDD rather than psychiatric disorder in general. The findings imply that strategies to interrupt ruminative processes may be helpful in minimizing persistence of first episode MDD in adolescence.

In 2004 Prospective Study of Rumination and Depression in Early Adolescence was done by Patricia C. Broderick, Constance Korteland. In this study, rumination, depression, and gender role were measured in a group of fourth through sixth graders once each year for 3 years. Results supported the primary hypothesis that rumination level would best predict level of depression at each subsequent assessment. No differences were observed between genders on depression or rumination. However, masculine and feminine-identified adolescents had higher depression scores than androgynous individuals, and feminine identified adolescents had the highest rumination scores overall. Links between rumination, depression, inability to distract, and gender role are explored, and possible treatments are discussed

Authors Jay K. Brinker and David J.A. Dozois wrote an article on Ruminative thought style and depressed mood in 2008 Recent research has suggested that the measure most commonly used to assess rumination, the Response Style Questionnaire (RSQ; L. D. Butler & S. Nolen-Hoeksema, 1994), may be heavily biased by depressive symptoms, thereby restricting the scope of research exploring this construct. This article offers a broader conceptualization of rumination, which includes positive, negative, and neutral thoughts as well as past and future-oriented thoughts. The first two studies describe the development and evaluation of the Ruminative Thought Style Questionnaire (RTS), a psychometrically sound measure of the general tendency to ruminate. Further, the scale is comprised of a single factor and shows high internal consistency, suggesting that rumination does encompasses the factors mentioned. The final study involved a longitudinal diary investigation of rumination and mood over time. Results suggest that the RTS assesses a related, but separate, construct than does the RSQ. RTS scores predicted future depressed mood beyond the variance accounted for by initial depressed mood whereas RSQ scores did not. The implications of these results and directions for future research are discussed.

Zia Lakdawalla et al. (2007) reviewed longitudinal studies examining three central cognitive theories of depression — Beck's theory, Hopelessness theory, and the Response Styles theory — among children (age 8–12) and adolescents (age 13–19). We examine the effect sizes in 20 longitudinal studies, which investigated the relation between the cognitive vulnerability–stress interaction and its association with prospective elevations in depression after controlling for initial levels of depressive symptoms. The results of this review suggest that across theories there is a small relation between the vulnerability–stress interaction and elevations in depression among children (pr = 0.15) and a moderately larger effect (pr = 0.22) among adolescents. Despite these important findings, understanding their implications has been obscured by critical methodological, statistical, and theoretical limitations that bear on cognitive theories of depression. The evidence base has been limited by poor measurement of cognitive vulnerabilities and over reliance on null hypothesis significance testing; these have contributed to a field with many gaps and inconsistencies.

Rumination in adolescents at risk for depression was the study done by Willem Kuyken et al. in 2006. This study examined the association between a hypothesized psychological vulnerability factor (rumination) and depression in adolescents. A behavioral high-risk design differentiated a sample of 326 adolescents (aged 14–18) as either at normal or high risk for depression (operationalzed as scores on a measure of neuroticism).Adolescents at risk for depression reported more rumination than adolescents not at risk. We hypothesized that the well established relationship between neuroticism and depression would be mediated by rumination in cross-sectional analyses, and our findings suggest that rumination partially mediated this relationship. The findings tentatively suggest that neuroticism acts as a risk factor for adolescent onset depression through increased tendency towards brooding rumination (i.e. moody self-evaluative dwelling) in response to depressed mood. Prospective and experimental research examining this mechanism is required.

Peter Muris et al. found the relationship between Rumination and Worry in Nonclinical Adolescents in 2004. They examined relationships between self-reported rumination as assessed by the Children's Response Style Scale (CRSS), worry as measured by the Penn State Worry Questionnaire for Children (PSWQ-C), and anxiety and depression symptoms as indexed by respectively the Screen for Child Anxiety Related Emotional Disorders (SCARED) and the Children's Depression Inventory (CDI) in a sample of 337 nonclinical adolescents aged 12–17 years. Results showed that rumination and worry were substantially correlated. Further, a factor analysis showed that both constructs were nevertheless distinct as rumination and worry items loaded on separate factors. Interestingly, both rumination and worry correlated more substantially with anxiety symptoms than with depression symptoms. Finally, worry emerged as a unique predictor of anxiety symptoms, even when controlling for rumination. In contrast, when controlling for worry, rumination no longer accounted for a significant proportion of the variance in depression symptoms.

Ruminative Thoughts and Their Relation to Depression and Anxiety was the title of study done by Jennifer A. Harrington and Virginia Blankenship in 2002. Although past research has shown a correlation between ruminative response style and depression (Nolen-Hoeksema, 1991), the basic relationships among amount of ruminative thoughts, depression, and anxiety has not been established. Scores from the Beck Depression Inventory-Second Edition (BDI-II; Beck, Steer, & Brown, 1996), the Beck Anxiety Inventory (BAI; Beck & Steer, 1993), and the McIntosh and Martin (1992) Rumination Scale were analyzed for 199 participants. The correlation between rumination and depression was .33, between rumination and anxiety was .32, and between depression and anxiety was .56. The partial correlation between rumination and depression (controlling for anxiety level) was .20, and the partial correlation between rumination and anxiety (controlling for depression level) was .17. The finding that rumination is not unique to depression but is also associated with the specific negative affect of anxiety alone might also suggest new treatments of these two prevalent disorders.

Effectiveness of group counseling

The literature supporting the effectiveness of group counseling in alleviating symptoms of depression and anxiety is vast. Due to the co morbidity of anxiety and depression, the group counseling literature tends to investigate them simultaneously. Therefore, this section will explore the two phenomena together.

Although some groups have been formed specifically to address symptoms of anxiety and depression, groups formed with other goals have also resulted in decreased symptoms of both anxiety and depression (Wang and Li, 2003; Biggam and Power, 2002; Pfeffer, Jiang, Kakuma, Hwang and Metsch, 2002; Hayward, 2000; Clarke, 1999; Lee and Hett, 1990). For instance, groups have been formed for the purpose of helping people who suffer from the consequences of addictions either directly or indirectly through the use of a family member or loved one (Kuhns, 1993; Freudenberger, 1990; Dittrich and Trapold, 1983). These groups often lead to a lessening of depression and anxiety in its group members.

Steven D. Hollon, Michael O. Stewart, and Daniel Strunk in 2016 found Enduring effect of cognitive behavior therapy in the treatment of depression and anxiety that reduce risk for subsequent symptom return following treatment termination. These enduring effects have been most clearly demonstrated with respect to depression and the anxiety disorders. It remains unclear whether these effects are a consequence of the amelioration of the causal processes that generate risk or the introduction of compensatory strategies that offset them and whether these effects reflect the mobilization of cognitive or other mechanisms. No such enduring effects have been observed for the psychoactive medications, which appear to be largely palliative in nature. Other psychosocial interventions remain largely untested, although claims that they produce lasting change have long been made. Whether such enduring effects extend to other disorders remains to be seen, but the capacity to reduce risk following treatment termination is one of the major benefits provided by the cognitive and behavioral interventions with respect to the treatment of depression and the anxiety disorders.

Turki Alotaibi in 2015 did an evidence-based review of the literature in order to provide new and innovative approaches to developing and improving student counseling skills, methods, and frameworks in order to directly combat anxiety and depression in Saudi schools. Non-empirical qualitative review of the literature on anxiety and depression and on student counselling in the United Kingdom and in Saudi Arabia. The research study argues that in theory student counsellors in Saudi schools can help to direct address and reduce the existing high prevalence of anxiety and depression in youths and adolescents attending Saudi schools. The research study concludes that student counselling in Saudi schools could potentially help in directly combating and reducing levels of anxiety and depression among Saudi school children and adolescents.

Comorbidity of Anxiety and Depression in Youth was found out by Jessica L. Schleider, Elizabeth D. Krause and Jane E. Gillhamin (2014). Their review synthesized current knowledge of relations between childhood anxiety and adolescent depression, focusing on the possibility that primary anxiety in childhood may cause secondary depression in adolescents. Across existing studies, evidence strongly supports childhood anxiety as a risk factor for adolescent depression, and long-term follow-up studies of cognitive behavioral childhood anxiety treatments may suggest a causal anxiety-depression link. However, mechanisms underlying this relationship remain unexplored. Future directions include careful assessment of comorbidity between anxiety and depressive disorders, longitudinal evaluations of anxiety and depression following interventions for childhood anxiety, and investigations of mediators and moderators of the anxiety-depression link. Finally, mechanisms by which the treatment of childhood anxiety might prevent depression in adolescents are proposed.

Horowitz *et al.* (2007) evaluated the efficacy of intervention programs for preventing depressive symptoms in adolescents. Participants were 380 high school students randomly assigned to a Cognitive Behavioral Program (CB), an Interpersonal Psychotherapy Adolescent Skill Training Program (IPT-AST) or a no-intervention control. The intervention involved eight 90 minutes weekly session run in small groups during wellness classes. At post intervention, students in both the CB and IPT-AST groups reported significantly lower levels of depressive symptoms than did those in the no intervention group.

Ramsay and Main (2007) utilized a quasi experimental pretest-post test design to assess the effectiveness of counselling type, in a sample of individuals diagnosed with low self esteem, high in anxiety and depression. Nine females underwent group peer counselling and nine underwent individual counselling. Both group peer counselling and individual counselling are found to significantly increasing self-esteem, self reported levels of overall life satisfaction and reduced anxiety and depression.

An evaluation of the effectiveness of Cognitive Behaviour Therapy for 12-14 year old school children was done by Habib, Seif (2007). The sample comprised 198 boys and 136 girls. Students were assessed using the Child Depression Inventory and the Coopersmith Self-Esteem Inventory. The 32 children with depression were offered Cognitive Behavior Therapy. They were assessed 3 months after the intervention using the same tools and the results indicate the effectiveness of this therapy and reduction in depressive symptoms.

Eric Stice Emily Burton., Sarah Kate Bearman and Paul Rohde in 2006 did a randomized trial on depression prevention. This trial compared a brief group cognitive–behavioral (CBT) depression prevention program to a waitlist control condition and four placebo or alternative interventions. High-risk adolescents with elevated depressive symptoms (N=225, M age = 18, 70% female) were randomized to CBT, supportive–expressive group intervention, bibliotherapy, expressive writing, journaling, or waitlist conditions and completed assessments at baseline, termination, and 1- and 6-month follow-up. All five active interventions showed significantly greater reductions in depressive symptoms at termination than waitlist controls; effects for CBT and bibliotherapy persisted into follow-up. CBT, supportive–

expressive, and bibliotherapy participants also showed significantly greater decreases in depressive symptoms than expressive writing and journaling participants at certain follow-up points. Findings suggest there may be multiple ways to reduce depressive symptoms in high-risk adolescents, although expectancies, demand characteristics, and attention may have contributed to the observed effects.

School-based prevention of depression and anxiety symptoms in early adolescence: A pilot of a parent intervention component by Gillham, Jane E et al. in 2006. This pilot study investigated the effectiveness of a cognitive-behavioral depression prevention program, the Penn Resiliency Program for Children and Adolescents (the PRP-CA), when combined with a parent intervention component. Forty-four middle school students and their parents were randomly assigned to the enhanced PRP (the PRP-CA plus parent program) or control conditions. Students completed measures of depression and anxiety symptoms at baseline and 2 weeks, 6 months, and 1 year after the intervention ended. The combined version of the PRP significantly reduced symptoms of depression and anxiety during the follow-up period. Children assigned to the intervention condition were less likely than controls to report clinical levels of anxiety symptoms. Findings suggest that school-based cognitive-behavioral interventions that include parents may prevent depression and anxiety symptoms in early adolescence.

Martin E.P. Seligman, Peter Schulman and Alyssa M. Tryon in 2006 did study on Group prevention of depression and anxiety symptoms. For this they delivered a brief, classroom-based cognitive-behavioral workshop along with ongoing Web-based materials and e-mail coaching to college students at risk for depression. At risk was defined as having mild to moderate depressive symptoms on a self-report measure of depression. Two hundred forty students were randomized into either an eight-week workshop that met in groups of 10, once per week for 2 h or into an assessment-only control group. They plan to track participants for 3 years after the workshop and here we report the 6 month preventive effects on depression and anxiety. The workshop group had significantly fewer depressive symptoms and anxiety symptoms than the control group, but there was no significant difference between the conditions on depression or anxiety episodes at 6 month follow up. The workshop group had significantly better well being than the control group, and the workshop group had significantly greater improvement in optimistic explanatory style than the control group. Improved explanatory style was a significant mediator of the prevention effects from pre- to post-workshop for depressive and anxiety symptoms, as well as for improved well being.

Researchers posited that group counseling can be helpful in alleviating depression and anxiety in psychotic patients. Warman, Grant, Sullivan, Caroff, and Beck (2005) conducted a study involving group therapy with six patients with positive symptoms of psychosis. The group met for 12 weeks, and their levels of depression, anxiety, stress, and hopelessness were assessed before and after treatment and again at an 11-month follow-up. The results showed a significant decrease in participants' levels of depression, anxiety, and hopelessness. Additionally, the majority of the gains were maintained over an 11-month follow-up period. The authors concluded that group therapy may offer benefits for patients with psychosis in terms of less delusional thinking, and lower levels of depression and anxiety when used as an adjunctive treatment.

A characteristic of group counseling is that the group is formed around a concern that is common to all members. An example of this is a chronic illness. Because those who suffer from chronic illness often suffer from psychological distress, the process of group counseling often helps participants' depression and anxiety. For instance, several groups have been formed for individuals who have cancer. Aguero-Trotter (2005) examined the effects of a coping skills training group and a support group on cancer patients' levels of distress, coping and adjustment to cancer, depression, and anxiety. The participants were randomly assigned to one of the two treatment groups: support group or coping skills training. The groups met for 8 weekly two-hour session. Emotional distress, coping, psychological adjustment, depression, and anxiety were assessed before and after the intervention via survey. The results indicated that the participants in the skills training group had significantly lower levels of distress. However, both groups produced lower levels coping, psychosocial adjustment, anxiety, and depression. The authors concluded that both support group and skills training have the potential to help people suffering from cancer.

Stress, Anxiety, Depression, And Loneliness Of Graduate Counseling Students: The Effectiveness Of Group Counseling And Exercise by Jonna Lynn Byars (2005). This study examined the effectiveness of group counseling and exercise in alleviating the symptoms of stress, anxiety, depression, and loneliness in graduate counseling students. Participants in this study self-selected into one of three treatment groups: exercise, group counseling, or control. All participants were enrolled in a master's level counseling class in a CACREP accredited program. A total of 57 graduate students participated in this study; 17 were in the group counseling treatment group, 19 were in the exercise treatment group, and 21 were in the control treatment group.

Participants in the group counseling group met for 1.5 hours per week for 10 weeks and participated in group counseling led by a doctoral level counselor. Participants in the exercise group exercised for 45 minutes twice per week for 10 weeks. Participants in the control group received no treatment for 10 weeks. This study utilized a quasi-experimental nonrandomized pretest/posttest design. MANCOVA was used to test for significance among the groups. The following instruments were employed at both pretest and posttest: (1) the Beck Depression Inventory, (2) the Beck Anxiety Inventory, (3) the Perceived Stress Scale, and (4) the UCLA Loneliness Scale. Results of this study indicate both group counseling and exercise significantly reduce the symptoms of stress, anxiety, and depression in graduate counseling students as compared to the control group. No significant differences were found between the effectiveness of group counseling and exercise in alleviating symptoms of anxiety, stress, and depression in graduate counseling students. Results also suggest that group counseling is effective for alleviating symptoms of loneliness in graduate counseling students as compared to no treatment and exercise treatment. A comparison of the results of this study to previous research is provided, along with implications of this research for training, practice, and future research.

Similar to Warman et al. (2005), the author concluded that group psychotherapy is a helpful adjunct to treatment for people who suffer from psychosis. Group counseling has also been found to be helpful in a nonresearch community setting. Peterson and Halstead (1998) investigated the effectiveness of group cognitive behavioral therapy for 138 adult patients referred by mental health clinics two- hour depression management groups extending for six weeks. Patients were assessed before and after by the Beck Depression Inventory (BDI). Groups consisted of six to nine randomly assigned participants. The results showed that level of depression was significant decreased by 64% of the participants, the average reduction was 38%, and 43% had a greater than 50% reduction in their BDI scores. The results indicated that group therapy can be effectively applied in a clinical setting with a heterogeneous patient population. The authors concluded that group therapy is a cost-effective treatment approach and the potential for its benefits significantly outweighs the costs. Additionally, the authors wrote "In this era of managed care initiatives, group cognitive behavioral therapy for depression should be considered as first-line treatment intervention for many patients with depression as part of a stepped-care treatment approach to provide the best treatment at the best value"

Solution-Focused Brief Therapy was the result of a social aid worker's efforts namely Steve De Shazer (2005) and his co-workers in MRI family health center located in Milwaukee (Goldenberg & Goldenberg, 2000). This attitude focuses on difficult exceptions; from this point of view, changes and revolutions are inevitable affairs; especially possible positive changes. So in this kind of treatment, the focus is on affairs which have potential of a change rather than on difficult aspects which cannot be changed (Hanlon, O & Weiner-Davis, M 1989 cited by Nazari & Nawabinijad, 2006, Nazari & Goli, 2007). So this treatment is well-known as Hope Consultation (Nunnlly, 1993).

Various age groups have been helped by group counseling. These include college age, children, and seniors. With regards to college age, Wang and Li (2003) examined the effect of eight, 1.5 hour sessions of group counseling on levels of self-confidence in 15 college students. The effects of the group were assessed before and after the treatment by the Symptom Checklist (SCL-90) and the 16 Personality Factor (16 PF) Questionnaire. The results showed the scores of interpersonal relationships, anxiety, and compulsiveness of the SCL-90 significantly reduced while the factors scores of emotion stability, adaptation, independence, and personality of the 16 PF improved. The authors concluded that group counseling can help college students to improve interpersonal relationships, raise self-confidence, lower anxiety, and encourage communication.

Trozzolino (2003) evaluated the effectiveness of a 12-week psychoeducational group in improving mood and glycemic control in adults with diabetes and visual impairments. In this study, the 48 participants were randomly assigned to one of two groups: the experimental group (group treatment) and the control group (no treatment). All participants were administered the following three psychometric tests before and after the 12 week treatment period: the Beck Depression Inventory, the Michigan Diabetes Knowledge Test, and the Problem Areas in Diabetes Survey (PAID). The results showed that the participants in the psychoeducational group counseling made statistically significant gains in glycemic control as compared to the control group, and there was a significant positive relationship between glycemic control and depression. This means those who participated in the group not only were not only better able to control their illness, but also had fewer symptoms of depression. Group counseling has also been helpful for family members' of persons with chronic illness. Pomeroy (1995) investigated the effectiveness of group counseling for 33 family members of people with AIDS. The participants underwent an eight-week psychoeducational and task-centered group that met for 1.5 hours per week. The participants were assessed before and after treatment via questionnaire on their levels of stress, depression, perceived stigma, and anxiety. The results showed that group counseling significantly reduced family members of people with AIDS levels of stress, depression, and anxiety.

Similar to the study by Freudenberger, several investigations have been conducted to examine the effect group counseling has on adolescents' symptoms of anxiety and depression. For instance, Biggam and Power (2002) compared the effectiveness of a 10 week, group-based problem solving intervention with a no-treatment wait list control group. The 46 participants were young (16-21 years old) incarcerated offenders and randomly assigned to either the group intervention or control. Participants' levels of anxiety, depression, hopelessness, and their social problem-solving were assessed via questionnaire before and after the treatment. Results indicated that the participants in the group counseling intervention experienced significant reductions in their levels if anxiety, depression, and hopelessness; and improvement in their self assessment. The authors concluded that group counseling is a helpful adjunct to treatment for incarcerated adolescents.

With regards to children, Pfeffer, Jiang, Kakuma, Hwang and Metsch (2002) evaluated the efficacy of group counseling for children who suffered suicide of a parent or sibling. The 75 participants, aged 6-15 years old, were randomly assigned either to receive (39 children) or not to receive (36 children) the treatment. The group treatment consisted of 10 weekly sessions, lasting 1.5 hours and each group, and had two to five children of similar development levels in each group. The following instruments were used at the initial and outcome assessments: Schedule for Affective Disorders and Schizophrenia for School- Age Children, Beck Depression Inventory,

Childhood Posttraumatic Stress Reaction Index, Children's Depression Inventory, Revised Children's Manifest Anxiety Scale, and the Social Adjustment Inventory for Children and Adolescents. The results showed that the children who received the group treatment had a significant decrease in anxiety and depressive symptoms, as compared to the control group. The authors concluded that bereavement group counseling focusing on reactions to death and suicide and strengthening coping skills can lessen distress, anxiety, and depression in children after parental or sibling suicide.

Another group of individuals suffering from a chronic illness that has been helped by group counseling is individual suffering from psoriasis. Dowling (2002) examined qualitative responses from women with psoriasis who participated in short-term, time limited group psychotherapy that utilized Yalom's (1995) psychotherapy approach. The 11 participants participated in a 10-week group that met for 1 hour per week. The researcher investigated the psychological consequences of psoriasis (anxiety, depression, self-esteem, and quality of life) in relation to some psychological predictors of adjustment to psoriasis. The author provided a comprehensive qualitative analysis of participant responses and group changes by assessing changes in both individual group members and the group as whole by focusing on the presence, absence, and changes in Yalom's therapeutic factors. The data revealed that group participation was beneficial to all members. Participants became more cognizant of how they relate to others, learned new coping skills, and developed a better understanding of the importance of social support. Most group members indicated one or more of the following benefits: decreased feelings of anxiety and depression; an increase in quality of life and feelings of selfesteem; and a greater ability to cope. The author concluded that this study provides support of group counseling for people with psoriasis and acknowledges the significance of the group process itself. Individuals diagnosed with diabetes experiencing low vision have also been helped by group counseling.

Hayward (2000) conducted a similar study that compared the efficacy of cognitive behavioral group therapy to a control wait list treatment group in adolescents. The participants in this study were 35 female adolescent with social phobia who were randomly assigned to either the treatment or control group. The treatment consisted of 16 cognitive behaviorally based group treatment sessions that were 1.5 hours in duration. The participants were assessed prior to and following the 16 week treatment period by the Social Phobia and Anxiety Inventory and the Anxiety Disorders Interview Schedules. The results indicated that the group treatment produced a significant reduction in symptoms of anxiety. Additionally, it was noted that a significant number of participants in the group no longer met the DSM-IV criteria for social phobia. The author further noted that for participants with a history of major depression, treatment for social phobia reduces the risk for relapse of major depression

Similarly, Boll (1998) investigated short-term group psychotherapy for seven individuals diagnosed with schizophrenia. The group met for 12 weekly, 90-minute sessions. The participants were assessed qualitatively with clinical observations, client verbalizations, and the Patients' Ranking Statements Questionnaire before and after treatment. The qualitative analysis revealed the clients showed significant improvement in coping with delusions and hallucination, social skills, interpersonal relationships, and social anxiety.

Similar to the previous study by Haward, Clarke (1999) investigated the effectiveness of cognitive-behavioral therapy (CBT) group counseling on adolescents. However, in this study, both acute and maintenance effects on depression were examined. The 126 participants, who were between 14 and 18 years old and met the DSM-III diagnosis of major depression or dysthymia, were randomly assigned to one of three eight-week acute treatment conditions: (1) adolescent group CBT (16 two-hour sessions, adolescent-only); (2) adolescent CBT with a separate parent group (16 two-hour sessions, adolescent-parent); or (3) wait list control. Subsequently, participants completing the acute CBT were randomly assigned to one of three conditions for the 24-month follow-up period: (1) assessments every 4 months with booster sessions; (2) assessments only every four months; or (3) assessments only every 12 months. The following assessments were administered before treatment, following the acute phase and during the assessments in the 24-month follow-up period: Schedule for Affective Disorders ad Schizophrenia for School-Age Children, longitudinal Interval Follow-up Evaluation, and the Beck Depression Inventory. The participants' parents completed the Child Behavior Checklist at the assessment points. Of the 126 initial participants, 96 completed the entire treatment. Results showed that the acute CBT groups produced higher depression recovery rates than the waitlist. Outcomes for the adolescent-only and adolescent-parent conditions were not significantly different. Rates of recurrence during the two-year follow-up were lower than found with treated adult depression. The booster sessions did not reduce the rate of recurrence during the follow-up period, but did accelerate recovery in participants who were still depressed after the acute phase. The authors concluded that the findings support the effectiveness of group therapy in alleviating adolescent depression.

In a similar study, Evans (1995) investigated the effects of cognitive-behavioral and socially supportive group therapy on depressed cancer patients. Seventy-two depressed cancer patients were randomly assigned to one of three treatment conditions: cognitive-behavioral group therapy (29 participants), support group therapy (23 participants), or no-treatment control condition (20 participants). The groups met for onehour weekly sessions for eight weeks, and each group contained six to nine participants. All participants were assessed before and after treatment and at a six-month follow-up via the following questionnaires: the Center for Epidemiological Studies Depression Scale, the Social Provisions Scale, Symptom Checklist, and the Multidimensional Health Locus of Control Scale. The results indicated that the depressed patients who received brief group therapy intervention exhibited greater reduction in emotional distress than members of a comparison group who did not participate in a group intervention. Although both the cognitive-behavioral and social support group interventions produced significant reductions in depression, anxiety, and somatization, the social support group intervention also resulted in a significant reduction in overall post-intervention psychiatric symptoms, as well as significantly less somatic preoccupation, anxiety, and depression at follow-up. The author concluded both forms of group therapy lessen symptoms of distress for depressed cancer patients, with the support groups demonstrating longer lasting change.

As with children and adolescents the elderly have also profited from group counseling. Ladish (1993) investigated the efficacy of cognitive behavioral therapy and support group treatment on 22 moderately to severely depressed elderly participants. All participants were randomly assigned to one of the two treatment groups for 12 weeks. Pre-and post-treatment data was gathered via survey to assess levels of depression, coping, and support. The researcher reported that significant time effects for both treatments while interaction effects comparing treatments across time were not significant. Symptoms of depression, coping, and support all showed high levels of improvement in both groups. The author concluded both cognitive behavioral group therapy and support groups are helpful at alleviating elderly patient's symptoms of depression.

Kuhns (1993) investigated the effectiveness of dynamic group psychotherapy and self-help groups for college-aged adult children of alcoholics. In the quasi-experimental pretest posttest design, the 150 participants (75 who were alcoholics and 75 who were not raised by alcoholics) were randomly assigned to one of four groups: (a) 25 alcoholics who received an 11 week treatment of self-help support group therapy; (b) 25 alcoholics who received an 11 week treatment of dynamic group psychotherapy; (c) 25 alcoholics who were a control group and received no treatment; and (d) 75 college-aged children of non-alcoholic parents who were a control group. All participants were administered the pretest which consisted of the Tennessee Self-Concept Scale which measured self-concept, the Coping Resource Inventory Scale which measured coping behaviors, and the Center for Epidemiologic Studies Depression Scale which measured levels of depression. After the 11 weeks of treatment, or no treatment for the control groups, posttests of the same instruments were administered. The results indicated that the alcoholics had lower self-concepts, fewer coping behaviors, and higher levels then children from non-alcoholic families.

Another study to examine the effectiveness of group counseling and depression in those affected by addiction was conducted by Freudenberger (1990). This study investigated the effectiveness of group psychotherapy on 50 adolescent boys (mean age, 19.2 years) who were poly-substance users with long histories of drug abuse. The participants were administered following four scales: the Substance Abuse Problem Checklist, Multiscore Depression Inventory, State Trait Inventory, and Tennessee Self- Concept before and after undergoing 15 weeks of treatment. The results showed that the group psychotherapy significantly reduced levels of depression and state and trait anxiety. Additionally, the participants' self-concepts were improved and motivations for treatment were enhanced. The authors concluded that group psychotherapy can provide those who suffer from addictions help at alleviating both anxiety and depression.

Individuals experiencing a major life transition have also been helped by group counseling. Lee and Hett (1990) investigated the effectiveness of group counseling for people who were recently divorced. The participants were 12 adults who had divorced within the past six months and 12 waiting-list controls. The group met for eight weekly sessions for 1.5 hours each session. Participants were assessed via questionnaire before and after the 12-week treatment period. The results indicated that the group intervention promoted a significant decrease in depression and anxiety, an increased ability to live in the present, greater independence, more spontaneity, and an increase in experimental participants' ability to form meaningful relationships. The authors noted that group counseling should be considered a very helpful and cost-effective treatment for people going through a divorce.

Another study that involved addictions was conducted by Dittrich and Trapold (1983). In this investigation, the effectiveness of brief group treatment aimed at ameliorating some of the psychological reactions commonly seen in the wives of alcoholics was explored. Prior to and after the 8 week treatment, the 10 participants' levels of anxiety, self-concept, depression, and enabling behaviors were assessed via questionnaire and compared to a waiting list control group. The participants in the brief group therapy treatment showed significant improvement in anxiety, self-concept, and enabling behaviors; there was no initial difference in depression. After the formal treatment, the experimental group was given access to a support group which met for the next eight weeks and was again assessed with the same questionnaires. The wait list control group replicated the treatment sequence as it had been given to the original treatment group. An analysis of the experimental and control groups combined over the various treatment phases indicated significant improvements on measures of depression, anxiety, self-concept, and enabling at the end of the formal treatment. The authors concluded that not only were the group therapy and support groups helpful in alleviating depression and anxiety, but also that wives of alcoholics can be treated effectively for their psychological reactions independently of their husbands' treatment.

School-based interventions

Schools are an ideal venue to provide empirically supported treatments to children. Children spend a large amount of time at school, making it an easy child accessible setting. Because of this, parents need not have scheduling conflicts around school and work schedules, and it eliminates any transportation difficulties or needs. Also, private or community-based treatment can be costly, whereas school-based services are often free of charge or inexpensive. Moreover, mental health services have the potential to become one of the many routine educational services provided (i.e., speech and language therapy, occupational therapy, physical therapy, etc.). There is also some stigma around receiving mental health services. A natural setting such as a school might help alleviate the negative stigma and promote a more positive attitude about youth receiving mental health services.

School-based cognitive behavioral interventions for anxious youth: study protocol for a randomized controlled trial by Bente Storm Mowatt Haugland et al (2017). Anxiety disorders are prevalent among adolescents and may have long-lasting negative consequences for the individual, the family and society. Cognitive behavioral therapy (CBT) is an effective treatment. However, many anxious youth do not seek treatment. Low-intensity CBT in schools may improve access to evidence-based services. We aim to investigate the efficacy of two CBT youth anxiety programs with different intensities (i.e., number and length of sessions), both group-based and administered as early interventions in a school setting. The objectives of the study are to examine the effects of school-based interventions for youth anxiety and to determine whether a less intensive intervention is non-inferior to a more intensive intervention. The present study is a randomized controlled trial comparing two CBT interventions to a waitlist control group. A total of 18 schools participate and we aim to recruit 323 adolescents (12-16 years). Youth who score above a cutoff on an anxiety symptom scale will be included in the study. School nurses recruit participants and deliver the interventions, with mental health workers as co-therapists and/or supervisors. Primary outcomes are level of anxiety symptoms and anxiety-related functional impairments. Secondary outcomes are level of depressive symptoms, quality of life and general psychosocial functioning. Non-inferiority between the two active interventions will be declared if a difference of 1.4 or less is found on the anxiety symptom measure post-intervention and a difference of 0.8 on the interference scale. Effects will be analyzed by mixed effect models, applying an intention to treat procedure. The present study extends previous research by comparing two programs with different intensity. A brief intervention, if effective, could more easily be subject to large-scale implementation in school health services.

A study titled as Anxiety Disorders and School-Based Treatments: Assessing School Pyschologists' Knowledge and Perceptions was done by Kelly A. Myhasuk (2014). Anxiety disorders are common in children and youth. Despite high prevalence rates, most children with anxiety disorders do not receive treatment. In fact, for the few children who are receiving treatment, schools are the primary source of mental health care. When left untreated, children experience significant disruptions in their academic, social, emotional, and behavioral functioning. Therefore, it is important for those working in schools to recognize and treat children with anxiety disorders. The present study surveyed school psychologists ($n = 178$) to assess their knowledge about anxiety disorders and about empirically supported school-based treatments. Also, this study sought to investigate school psychologists' knowledge about many of the difficulties faced by children and youth with anxiety disorders. In addition, this study sough to gain an understanding of the referral and identification processes involving children with anxiety disorders in school and the types of services and supports available to students with anxiety disorders. Results of this study indicated that the majority of school psychologists are at least somewhat to very knowledgeable about most types of anxiety disorders and related educational difficulties, with doctoral level school psychologists being more knowledgeable. However, few school psychologists reported being very knowledgeable about empirically supported school-based treatments for anxiety disorders. Another major finding was that behavior consultation was the most frequently reported approach to address anxiety symptoms. Despite cognitive behavioral (CBT) therapy receiving the greatest support, empirically, as an effective treatment, very few schools offer CBT as a treatment option. Also, few school psychologists reported being very competent in the delivery of CBT principles and interventions.

Schools tend to be the primary setting where children display impairment and significant levels of anxiety Therefore, schools provide unique opportunities to provide treatment in real life settings, making the potential for generalizability of coping skills greater. Last and of greatest importance, schools are already the main entry point to mental health services (Burns et al., 1995). When working with anxious children, cognitive-behavioral therapy (CBT) and behavioral interventions have received the greatest empirical support for effectiveness (Huberty, 2008). CBT is an amalgamation of a behavioral approach (i.e., psycho-education, relaxation training, exposure tasks, role play, rewards) with cognitive information processing (cognitive restructuring, cognitive distortions, cognitive deficiencies). When working within a CBT model, there is an understanding that emotions and accompanying behaviors are the result of the connection between a given situation, a personal belief system, and thoughts about the event (Mennuti, Freeman & Christner, 2006).

A considerable amount of attention has been given to empirically-supported, school based treatments. Evidence-based practice is a common term used to describe services that are based on sound theoretical principles and interventions supported through empirically based studies (Mennuti, Freeman & Christner, 2006). Almost two decades ago, one of the first randomized clinical trials found that CBT was efficacious for treating children with anxiety disorders (Kendall, 1994). Results indicated that children who participated in the 16-week CBT treatment (Coping Cat) had significant reductions in anxious symptoms and/or no diagnosable anxiety disorder following treatment, compared with the waitlist control group. In addition, the children who received the CBT treatment maintained the treatment gains after a one year follow-up. The intervention used in this study, Coping Cat, is a 16-session cognitive behavioral intervention used to treat children with anxiety disorder, specifically generalized anxiety disorder, social phobia, and separation anxiety in children and young adolescents (Kendall & Hedtke, 2006). Its overall goal is to teach children to recognize signs of anxiety and to let these serve as cues to use the coping and anxiety management strategies taught in treatment.

Using a modular CBT approach in a school setting, Chiu et al. (2013) found that 95% of children who received the modular CBT demonstrated a positive treatment response by the end of treatment and were free of any anxiety diagnosis. In comparison, at the end of a 3-month waitlist, only 16.7% of children demonstrated a positive treatment response.

Positive Psychology at School: A School-Based Intervention to Promote Adolescents' Mental Health and Well-Being by Anat Shoshani and Sarit Steinmetz (2013). The present study evaluated a positive psychology school-based intervention aimed at enhancing mental health and empowering the entire educational staff and students at a large middle school in the center of Israel. 537 seventh- to ninth-grade students participated in a 1 year intervention program and were compared to 501 students in a demographically similar control school. In a 2-year longitudinal repeated measures design, the study assessed pre- to post-test modifications in psychological symptoms and distress and in targeted well-being factors that were promoted in the experimental but not in a wait list control condition. The findings showed significant decreases in general distress, anxiety and depression symptoms among the intervention participants, whereas symptoms in the control group increased significantly. In addition, the intervention strengthened self-esteem, self-efficacy and optimism, and reduced interpersonal sensitivity symptoms. These results demonstrate the potential benefits of evidence-based positive-psychology interventions for promoting school-children's mental health, and point to the crucial need to make education for well-being an integral part of the school curriculum.

Herzig-Andesrson, Colognori, Fox, Stewart, & Warner (2012) reviewed four school-based treatments for anxiety that have shown promise in controlled studies: Cool Kids, Baltimore Child Anxiety Treatment Study in the School (BCATSS), and Cognitive- Behavioral Intervention for Trauma in Schools (CBITS), and Skills for Academic Social Success (SASS). With the exception of the BCATSS which offers individual and group formats, the remaining interventions are intended to be used with groups and are grounded in CBT theory. Herzig-Anderson et al. (2012) found that each of these previously mentioned interventions had been supported with randomized control trials to demonstrate treatment efficacy and provided positive outcomes to anxious youth.

The effectiveness of a computer-assisted cognitive behavioral therapy program, Camp Cope-A-Lot (CCAL), was examined with anxious youth. CCAL is adapted from the already empirically support Coping Cat program. Khanna & Kendall (2010) found that children receiving CBT showed marked improvement, compared with those children in the control. However, the children in the computer assisted group showed the greatest improvement. Eighty-one percent of children in the computer-assisted CBT group no longer met criteria for their anxiety disorders, compared with 70% of children in the individual CBT group. Furthermore, higher levels of child satisfaction were reported from children in the computer-assisted CBT group. In other words, children receiving CCAL enjoyed the program and made better gains.

In addition to the manualized CBT interventions, modular CBT has demonstrated impressive results for supporting and treating youth with anxiety disorders. Modular means that it breaks complex activities into smaller parts that function independently (Friedberg, McClure & Hillwig Garcia, 2009). Here, the therapist has the flexibility to group together the empirically-supported techniques that have the same therapeutic purpose, which allows for the individual child's needs to be met.

Teachers and parents learn how to recognize symptoms of anxiety and develop skills that can be used with anxious children. This is important because children with anxiety disorders tend to go unnoticed (Layne, Bernstein, & March, 2006; Schoenfeld & Janney, 2008).

A study on the Effects of Group Counseling on Adolescent was done by Stress Melissa I. Kurlan (2007).The purpose of this study was to determine whether or not psycho-educational group counseling in the school relieves stress among adolescent students identified as experiencing excessive stress. This study also examined gender differences in the severity and types of stress and response to the counseling intervention. Two separate groups (male and female) of 6-8 sixth grade students participated in ten weeks of structured group counseling that took place during the school day and focused on stress and coping. The results indicated that group counseling does indeed reduce stress among adolescents of both genders, although there were some gender differences in the character of response. The study also found that there was no major difference in the total amount of stress symptoms reported by males and females, although there were gender differences in specific types of stress symptoms reported. Thus, psycho-educational group counseling conducted in the school setting appears to be a useful intervention for reducing stress among adolescent students. Male and female students do show some differences in the quality of stress reported and in the response to counseling.

Conjoint behavioral consultation offers some advantages over some of the traditional treatments models. Because parents and teachers are active members in the treatment process, they learn valuable skills that can then be used with other children. As a result, the skills they learn can be generalized to other children in the future, which make these services more cost-effective. Moreover, the mental health needs often are greater than the availability of services. With a consultation approach, the consultees have the ability to reach and deliver services to a greater number of children, compared with that of a sole consultant. With regard to anxiety disorders, the conjoint behavioral consultation can be very beneficial. Parents and teachers are more than treatment participants. In this model, they receive ongoing training, professional development, and guidance that make them intervention agents (Auster, Feeney-Kettler & Kratochwill, 2006). In addition to CBT, consultation, particularly conjoint behavioral consultation, can be used to promote the incorporation of empirically-supported school-based treatments for anxiety disorders (Auster, Feeney-Kettler, & Kratochwill, 2006).

Conjoint behavioral consultation includes parents and teachers in the consultation process. In this particular model, a clinician serves as the consultant and uses problem-solving strategies to address the needs of the consultees (parent and teacher) and client (student). In other words, the parent and teacher are joint consultees and the provision of consultation services provided to the school and family are mutually involved (Sheridan & McCurdy, 2005).

Deno (2005) outlines and describes the steps of problem-solving strategies used in consultation. First, in the problem identification stage, the consultant and the child's parents and teachers identify and prioritize their concerns for the child. Second, the problem definition phase, aims to provide an operational definition of the behaviors of concern and to create a treatment goal. The third stage is designing the intervention. In this stage, all parties work collaboratively to design a feasible intervention, which includes a plan for data collection and specific guidelines for implementation. The fourth stage is the intervention implementation, which includes delivering the intervention, collecting data, and monitoring treatment fidelity. The final step includes treatment evaluation. At this time, the consultant and consultees review the effectiveness of the intervention and decide if treatment goals have been met.

Chorpita, Taylor, Francis, Moffitt, & Austin (2004) evaluated the initial efficacy of a modular approach to CBT for anxiety disorders in youth. Although only seven children completed the study, all seven children experienced clinically significant improvement, with all principal diagnoses being absent post treatment and also after a six month follow-up.

Taking all the information together, CBT as a whole shows the potential for effective school-based treatment for anxious youth. However, one of its most highly scrutinized shortcomings is that treatments rely heavily on mental health clinicians to deliver the intervention, which is costly and resource intensive.

Another promising CBT intervention is FRIENDS, a family-based group CBT. Shortt, Barrett & Fox (2001) were the first to conduct a randomized clinical trial evaluating the efficacy of the FRIENDS program. Results indicated that 69% of children who completed the program were diagnosis-free post-treatment, compared with the waitlist control group. Furthermore, after a one year follow-up, 68% of the children who received treatment no longer met criteria of an anxiety disorder.

In addition, some researchers have found conjoint behavioral consultation to be quite effective for treating anxiety disorders. For example, Gortmaker, Warnes & Sheridan (2004) reported success in treating a boy with selective mutism using a conjoint behavioral consultation service delivery model. Prior to intervention, the young boy produced zero vocalizations while at school. By the end of the problem solving steps, the boy was able to produce an average of 7.7 vocalizations a day that were generalized to multiple people.

In a larger random clinical trial, very similar results were obtained. After receiving the Coping Cat treatment, children with anxiety disorders were found to benefit from the intervention, compared with the waitlist control group (Kendall et al., 1997). In fact, more than 50% of children no longer met diagnostic criteria for an anxiety disorder post-treatment, and therapeutic gains were maintained after a one year follow-up.

Although various CBT interventions and behavioral consultation have been shown to help children with anxiety, a review of the literature has shown that most interventions that demonstrated effectiveness were delivered by a mental health clinician. Because the cost of hiring mental health professionals may not be feasible for all schools, there is a significant need for effective school-based interventions for anxiety disorders to be delivered by school personnel Therefore, school psychologists may be the ideal candidate to implement these interventions.

A number of studies have demonstrated that anxiety and depression prevention programmes provided as universal or indicated interventions can be effective in the short-term when compared to no intervention groups. Few studies have compared the effectiveness of prevention programmes against other active interventions and where they have been reported programme effects are typically non-significant. Long-term evaluations are lacking with most studies assessing symptom reduction and are therefore more accurately conceptualised as early intervention rather than primary prevention programmes designed to reduce the incidence of new cases. The variability in treatment effects between studies, including those using the same programmes, suggest that factors other than the specific programme content are important. The role of factors that moderate treatment effects such as child gender, age, ethnicity and symptom severity or factors which mediate them, for example, leader training and supervision, student engagement and leader delivery skills should be investigated. A further factor which is emerging as important in implementation studies is the compatibility of prevention programmes with the school culture and competing priorities. How they practically fit within a complex and full timetable have been identified as major obstacles that can impede effective delivery. In order to have a significant public health benefit evidence based prevention programmes need to be effective when delivered under diverse conditions in everyday settings.

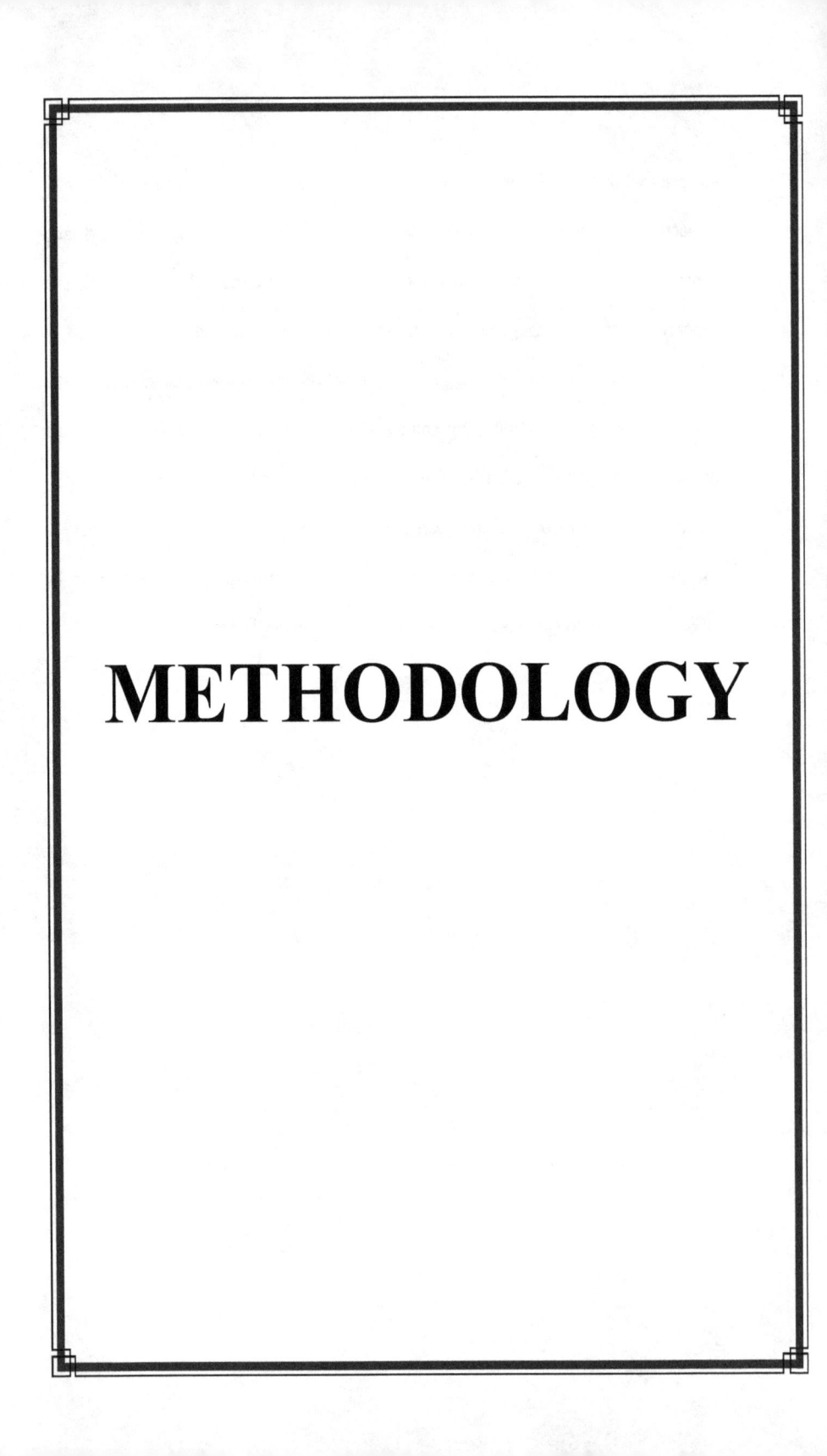

METHODOLOGY

METHODOLOGY

RATIONALE OF THE STUDY

In the recent years the Indian society seems to have undergone a total metamorphosis with changing roles of women, a breakdown of the joint family system, increased competitiveness in schools, increased sociability of the children, immense technological advances, peer and parental pressures resulting in an environment laden with stress and strain for the children. School counselors seem to have appeared like a blessing to the students and the parents to cope with the increased stress and strain and contribute towards maintaining the mental health of the younger generation. "School counseling is a profession that focuses on the relations and interactions between students and their school environment to reduce the effects of environmental and institutional barriers that impede student academic success. School counselors foster educational equity, access, and academic success in a rigorous curriculum to ensure that all students graduate from high school ready to succeed in college and careers. It is important for counselors to learn how they can better help students and to assess the effectiveness of their work. Group counseling is often a preference in schools because this approach can reach more students and is time effective. For this project the purposes of group involvement are to identify stressors that cause stress and anxiety, provide a forum for the discussion of these issues, and to teach students how to manage these things . It is the hope that through the group experience, students will gain an increased awareness of the stresses in their lives and increased coping skills.

"Adolescence" an age of turmoil and tribulations, a developmental transition period between childhood and adulthood often signals major physical, cognitive and socio-affective changes. It is considered a time of great stress or anxiety as it is marked by making decisions about who one is, who one want to be or how one wants to live his/her life. When levels of stress exceeds, it can lead to high level of anxiety or depression. Depression in high school or college 3–aged young people is not at all uncommon (Fleming & Offord, 1990). The corollary to this idea is that young people who experience episodes of depression during adolescence are at increasing risk for experiencing recurrences of depression during adulthood (Gotlib, Klein, Lewinsohn, Rohde & Seeley, 2000). Therefore, to preserve their psychological well-being and encourage their achievements, it is critical for students to be able to effectively deal with the stressful or negative events of their life.

While reviewing the researches it was found that counseling techniques proved to be important in treatment of anxiety, depression and stressful situations in adolescents. Therefore the present made an attempt to investigate the effect of counseling on anxiety and depression among adolescents.

OBJECTIVES

To compare the effectiveness of the group counseling in reducing anxiety and depression between the experiment pre and control pre groups.

To examine the effectiveness of the group counseling on optimism between the experimental pre and control pre groups.

To examine the impact of the group counseling on rumination between the experimental and control group in the pretest.

To compare the effectiveness of the group counseling intervention in reducing anxiety and depression between the experimental pre and control pre groups.

To examine the effectiveness of the group counseling on optimism between the experimental pre and control post groups.

To examine the impact of the group counseling on rumination between the experimental and control group in the post test conditions.

To investigate the efficacy of group counseling in reducing anxiety and depression in within group comparisons of experimental groups in pre-post test.

To examine the effect of group counseling on optimism in within group comparisons of experimental groups in pre-post test.

To examine the effect of group counseling on rumination in within group comparisons of control groups in pre-post test.

To investigate the efficacy of group counseling in reducing anxiety and depression in within group comparisons of control groups in pre-post test.

To examine the effect of group counseling on optimism in within group comparisons of control groups in pre-post test.

To examine the effect of group counseling on rumination in within group comparisons of control groups in pre-post test.

HYPOTHESES

There would be no significant difference in the level of depression and anxiety between the experimental and control groups in the pretest.

There would be no significant difference in optimism between the experimental and control groups in the pretest.

There would be no significant difference in rumination between the experimental and control groups in the pretest.

There would be a significant difference in the level of depression and anxiety between the experimental and control groups in the posttest after group counseling program.

There would be a significant difference in optimism between the experimental and control groups in the posttest.

There would be a significant difference in rumination between the experimental and control groups in the posttest.

There would be a significant difference in the level of depression and anxiety within group comparisons of experimental groups in pre-post test.

There would be a significant difference in optimism within group comparisons of experimental groups in pre-post test.

There would be a significant difference in rumination within group comparisons of experimental groups in pre-post test.

There would be no significant difference in the level of anxiety and depression in within group comparisons of control groups in pre-post test.

There would be no significant difference in the optimism within group comparisons of control groups in pre-post test.

There would be no significant difference in the rumination within group comparisons of control groups in pre-post test conditions.

VARIABLES

Independent Variable

Group Counseling program

Dependent Variables

Anxiety

Depression

Optimism

Rumination Response

RESEARCH DESIGN

The present study used pretest-posttest control group design. This design is used in such a way where one group (Experimental group) receives the treatment (X) ad another group (control group) receives no such treatment. As subjects are randomly assigned to the control group and the experimental group, the variables like selection and experimental mortality posing threats to internal validity are controlled.

R O1 X O2

R O3   O4

Where, R = population from which sample is being drawn, X = treatment given to the experimental group, O1 and O2 = experimental group pre and post treatment, O3 and O4 = control group pre and post conditions.

Table 3.1

PRE TEST (N =60)		TREATMENT GROUP COUNSELING INTERVENTION	POST TEST (N=60)	
Experimental Group (N = 30)	Control Group (N=30)		Experimental Group (N=30)	Control Group (N=30)
Depression	Depression		Depression	Depression
Anxiety	Anxiety		Anxiety	Anxiety
Optimism	Optimism		Optimism	Optimism
Rumination	Rumination		Rumination	Rumination

SAMPLE

The present study consisted of 400 adolescents of age group 13-18 years of a co-educational English medium school of Jaipur city. Non probability purposive sampling technique was used in the study. First the students were given suitable measure of measuring levels of depression and anxiety for screening. Out of 400, 60 students with high levels of depression and anxiety were selected. The selected sample was randomly divided into control and experimental group.

Inclusion criteria:

Age range: 13-18 years

Class: Class 9th -11th

Students of Co-ed English medium school

Depression scores ranging 21-40 (High scorers).

Anxiety scores ranging 22-35 (High scorers).

Not receiving treatment for any chronic/acute physical or mental illness.

Distribution of sample:

Table 3.2

S.No.	Characteristics	Experimental group	Control group
1.	No. of participants	30	30
2.	Gender distribution	Girls - 18 Boys - 12	Girls - 18 Boys - 12
3.	Age group	13-18 years	13-18 years

MEASURES

Demographic questionnaire

Demographic information of the participants was assessed using an information sheet that all participants completed prior to all measures of the proposed study. The information was related to name, age, gender, class, faculty, socio-economic status and educational status of the family, details of any physical illness, etc.

Beck's Depression Inventory

Depression levels were assessed with the Beck Depression Inventory (BDI, Beck, 1970), the most commonly used self-report measure of depression. The BDI is a Likert type scale that consists of 21 multiple choice items representing either a symptom or attitude related to depression.

Reliability and validity

Several studies have been conducted to establish the psychometric properties of the BDI (Beck, Epstein, Brown and Steer, 1988; Carter & Dacey, 1996; (Katz, Katz & Shaw, 1999; Skorikov & Vandervoort, 2003; Yin and Fan, 2000). For instance, Beck, Epstein, Brown, and Steer (1988) conducted a meta-analysis of 25 published papers using the BDI on individual diagnosed with schizophrenia, substance abuse, college students; and depressed students; the authors reported that reliabilities were consistently high, ranging from .73 to .95. Test-retest reliability for the scores on the BDI is stable for non-clinical populations, ranging from .70 to .90 for periods of 1 to 2 weeks (Beck & Steer, 118 1987). For psychiatric patients, test-retest reliability has been reported to range from .48 to .86 over various treatment periods (Katz, Katz & Shaw, 1999). Yin and Fan (2000) conducted a meta-analysis on the BDI and found results similar to those of Beck, Epstein, Brown, and Steer (1988). Yin and Fan investigated reliability coefficients for 1,200 research papers that have utilized the BDI. They found an overall mean reliability coefficient of .824, internal consistency of .837, and test-retest of .69. For different age ranges and study participants the internal consistency reliability coefficient were as follows: adolescent: .82; adult: .848; senior adult: .796; student participants: .835; nonstudent participants: .841; substance addicts: .769; nonsubstance addicts: .843. The test-retest reliability coefficients for different age ranges and study participants are as follows: adult: .67; senior adult: .862; physically ill: .630; normal .693; substance addicts: .587; non substance addicts: .713. In their investigation of the psychometric properties of the BDI with 261 undergraduate participants, Skorikov & Vandervoort (2003) found the BDI had a reliability of .86. Validity was established by correlating the BDI with the

Major Depression Subscale. Carter & Dacey (1996) investigated the validity of the BDI in 118 hospitalized adolescents. The adolescents were divided into two groups: 66 depressed patients and 52 nondepressed patients. The results indicated significant differences between the means of the two groups, thus establishing concurrent validity. Correlation coefficients among the BDI and MMPI-D were found to be significant, again supporting concurrent validity BDI scores have been shown to have concurrent validity. Beck et al. (1988) cited studies where correlations were reported between the BDI and other well-established instruments. These include the Hamilton Psychiatric Rating Scale (Hamilton, 1960),

Zung Self-Reported Depression Scale (Zung, 1965), the Multiple Affect Adjective Checklist Depression Scale (Zukerman & Lubin, 1965), and the clinicians' ratings of depth depression (Salkind, 1969). The correlations coefficients between the BDI and these other measures ranged from .59 to .96. The most significant relationship was found between the clinicians' ratings and the BDI where the correlation was reported at .96. Although, the BDI is useful for assessing many features of clinical depression, it does not provide enough information to establish a DSM diagnosis. The content validity of the BDI does assess for six of the nine DSM-IV-R criteria for a depressive episode; these are fatigue, insomnia, feelings of worthlessness, indecisiveness, suicide ideation, and loss of pleasure (Katz et al., 1999) The BDI does not assess for weight gain, hypersomnia, psychomotor agitation or retardation. Thus, the Beck Depression Inventory is best suited for assessing symptoms of depression, as it was in this study, not for diagnosing major depression.

Instructions

"Read each item carefully and circle the number next to the answer that best reflects how you have been feeling during the past few days. Make sure you circle one answer for each of the twenty-one (21) questions; if more than one answer applies, circle the highest number. Do not leave any questions unanswered."

Scoring and Interpretation:

Scores for each of the 21 questions were added by counting the number to the right of each marked question. The highest possible total for the whole test would be 63 and the lowest possible score is 0.

Table 3.3

Range of Scores	Interpretation
1-10	Normal
11-16	Mild mood disturbance
17-20	Borderline clinical depression
21-30	Moderate depression
31-40	Severe depression
Over 40	Extreme depression

Beck's Anxiety Inventory:

The Beck Anxiety Inventory (BAI, Beck & Steer, 1990) was used to assess symptoms of anxiety.

The Beck Anxiety Inventory is a 21-item, self-report instrument that assesses the overall severity of anxiety. Respondents are asked to rate the severity of each symptom using a 4-point scale ranging from (0) "Not at all bothered" to (3) "Severely bothered".

Reliability and Validity

With respect to reliability, several studies have demonstrated that the BAI serves as a reliable measure. The internal consistency of the BAI appears to be quite high with alphas ranging from .90 to .94 in both clinical and nonclinical samples at a variety of developmental stages (Beck, Epstein, Brown, & Steer, 1988; deBeurs, Wilson, Chambless, Goldstein, Feske, 1997; Fydrich, Dowdall, Chambless, 1992; Jolly, Aruffo, Wherry & Livingston, 1993; Kabakoff, Segal, Hersen, Van Hasselt, 1997; Steer, Kumar, Ranieri & Beck, 1995). Analysis of test-retest reliability in a 7- to 11-day period yielded correlations of .67 (Fydrich et al., 1992) and .75 (Beck et al., 1988); deBeurs et al. (1997) reported high test-retest reliability ($r = .83$) and stability over a 1-month period. Regarding validity, scores on the BAI have displayed concurrent validity with both other self-report measures of anxiety and clinical ratings of anxiety. For example, the correlation of the Hamilton Anxiety Rating Scale (HARS; Hamilton, 1959) with the BAI is .56, $p < .001$ (deBeurs et al., 1997). The BAI has also been found to correlate with the State and Trait scales of the State-Trait Anxiety Inventory (Form Y; Spielberger, 1983) at .47 ($p < .01$) (Spielberger, 1983) and .58 ($p < .001$), respectively (Kabakoff et al., 1997). Convergent validity of the BAI has also been established in adult clinical populations (Beck et al., 1988; deBeurs et al., 1997; Fydrich et al. 1992), adolescent psychiatric patients (Jolly et al., 1993;

Steer et al., 1995), older adult psychiatric patients (Kabakoff et al., 1997), and community samples (Borden, Peterson & Jackson, 1991; Creamer, Foran, Bell, 1995). In their investigation with 217 older adult outpatients, Kabakoff Segal & Hersen, Van Hasselt (1997) found that the BAI demonstrated high internal consistency with a Cronbach's coefficient alpha of .90. Discriminate validity was assessed by examining mean score differences between patients who meet criteria for an anxiety disorder diagnosis and patients who did not meet criteria. A significant mean total difference between patient with an anxiety disorder and those without was found. The BAI also demonstrated good factorial validity, with somatic anxiety and a subjective anxiety factor emerging. It was also found that the BAI can be useful as a quick screening instrument in detecting the presence of a current anxiety disorder. Fydrich, Dowdall, & Chambless (1992) investigated the psychometric properties of the BAI with two studies. In the first study, the test-retest reliability and internal consistency of the scale were examined with 40 outpatients having anxiety disorders. The BAI showed high internal consistency (Cronbach's alpha = .94) and reliability over an average time lapse of 11 days ($r = .67$). The second study was conducted on 71 outpatients with anxiety disorders to assess the convergent and divergent validity of the inventory. The participants completed the BAI, the State-Trait Anxiety Inventory, the Beck Depression Inventory, and Daily Diary Ratings of Anxiety and Depression. The BAI performed better on tests of convergent and discriminate validity than did the Trait Anxiety. The correlation between the BAI and Diary Anxiety was significantly higher than that between the BAI and the Diary Depression. As compared to the State-Trait

Instructions:

"Below is a list of common symptoms of anxiety. Please carefully read each item in the list. Indicate how much you have been bothered by that symptom during the past month, including today, by circling the number in the corresponding space in the column next to each symptom."

Scoring and Interpretation:

Summing the ratings for all of the 21 symptoms scores the Beck Anxiety Inventory (BAI) total scores can range from 0 to 63. According to the manual (Beck & Steer, 1990), The total score can be interpreted as follows:

Table 3.4

Range of scores	Interpretation
0-9	Normal anxiety
10-18	Mild to moderate anxiety
19-29	Moderate to severe anxiety
30-63	Severe anxiety

Life Orientation Test (Revised)-LOT-R

The Life Orientation Test (LOT) was developed to assess individual differences in generalized optimism versus pessimism. It was made to improve upon Carver and Scheier's (1985) original LOT. This measure has been used in a good deal of research on the behavioral, affective, and health consequences of the Optimism/Pessimism dimension. This measure, and its successor the LOT-R, have been used in a good deal of research on the behavioral, affective, and health consequences of this personality variable.

Reliability and validity:

Table 3.5

Item	Corrected item Scale correlation
1	.43
3	.48
4	.50
7	.63
9	.57
10	.56

Test Retest correlation was .68, .60, .56 and .79 respectively suggesting that LOT R is highly stable. Intern-scale correlation ranged from .43-.63 suggests that each item is partially measuring the same underlying construct. Internal validity using Cronbach's alpha has been found to be r= .78 and test-retest reliability after 28 months was reported to be r = .79 Convergent and discriminant validity have also been found between the LOT-R and other psychological constructs, such as depression, anxiety, and self-esteem inventories. When used in research studies, optimism has been divided into three groups based on a set range of LOT-R scores. For example: low optimists range from 6 to 13, medium optimists- 14 to 21 and high optimists- 22 to 30 (Harju & Bolen, 1998).

Instructions:

"Indicate your level of agreement with each of the item on a 5 point scale, using the response format, strongly disagree to strongly agree."

Scoring and Interpretation:

The test comprised of 10 statements. Items 3,7 and 9 prior to scoring (0=4)(1=3)(3=1)(4=0) were reverse scored and other items 1,3,4,7,9 and 10 were summed up to obtain an overall score. Items 2, 5,6 and 8 are filler items only. They are not scored as part of the revised scale. The minimum and maximum scores are to be as 6 and 30 respectively, higher score indicating high level of optimism.

Ruminative Response Scale

A short version of the Ruminative Response Scale (RRS) formed by (Treynor et al (2003), consists 10 items from the original list of 22 which was developed by Nolen-Hoeksema and Morrow (1991). This instrument was created to exclude items of the RRS that have been found to measure depressive symptomology, rather than rumination, in order to eliminate conceptual overlap (Treynor et al., 2003).

Reliability and Validity:

The scale was obtained by selecting the items that had the highest item-total correlations with the total score. The short version is highly correlated to the full version of the scale ($r = .90$) and has a high level of internal reliability (Cronbach's a = .85). Each item is scored on a 4-point Likert scale, ranging from 1 ("almost never") to 4 (almost always"). Treynor and her colleges (2003) described that all Reflection items were 'neutrally valenced' and described engaging in contemplation to alleviate negative mood (sample items include 'Write down what you are thinking and analyze it 'and 'Go someplace alone to think about your feelings'') whereas the items of the Brooding had negative connotation and described 'moody pondering' (sample items include 'Think "Why do I always react this way?" and 'Think "Why do I have problems other people don't have?"). The inter-item reliability of the Reflection subscale was .72 and the test-retest correlation was r = 60. For the Brooding subscale, coefficient alpha was .77 and the test retest correlation was r =. 62 (Treynor et al., 2003).

Instructions:

"People think and do many different things when they feel sad, blue or depressed. Please read each of the items below and indicate whether you never, sometimes, often or always think or do each one when you feel sad, down or depressed. Please indicate what you generally do, not what you think you should do."

1 = Never

2= Sometimes

3 = Often

4= Always

Scoring and Interpretation:

Each item is scored on a 4 point Likert scale, ranging from 1(never) to 4 (always). All 10 items were summed and total score for rumination was obtained. The higher the score the more will be the rumination.

PROCEDURE

The present study was divided into three phases:

Phase 1: PRE INTERVENTION PHASE

The sample of 400 adolescents of co-educational English medium school from Jaipur city was selected for the present study. The age of the sample ranged from 13-18 years. First of all suitable measures for measuring anxiety and depression were administered. Participants who scored higher on depression and anxiety (N=60) were divided into experimental and control group with N=30 in each group. These two groups were given two additional questionnaires for measuring their level of optimism and rumination.

Phase 2: INTERVENTION PHASE

For intervention, a two month group counseling program was specifically designed and administered on experimental group. Each session was of 45 minutes exempting the Sundays and school holidays. This group counseling program was inspired by FRIENDS program (Barrett, P. (2005), Coping cat, coping koala (Kendall, Philip C 1994), and worry busters (Marilyn Campbell 2006) etc. school based interventions used widely by psychologists to work on adolescents' depression and anxiety specifically.

DETAILED DESCRIPTION OF THE GROUP COUNSELING PROGRAM

"GROUP SORTING"

The random distribution of the participants (N=60) into experimental and control group was done. Each group has 30 participants. The process was explained to both of the group in details in order to clear any doubts or query asked.

"RAPPORT BUILDING"

Rapport building was done with the participants by explaining the process of the intervention and playing ice breaking activity with them.

Objective: - To make the students interact with each other as there were different age groups present in the group. Having a little fun, get to know the group and making all age groups comfortable with each other so that further no awkwardness is there within group. Activity: - Scavenger Hunt was played with the participants.

Appendix 1

"GROUP COUNSELING SESSION -1"

Objective: - To have participants talk about their view of depression and to give them an introduction of exactly what depression is.

About "Depression"

- ❖ What is depression? What does it mean to be depressed?
- ❖ Taking in the views shared by the group and making them understand the concept of depression

Figure 3.1

<u>HOW WE UNDERSTAND DEPRESSION</u>

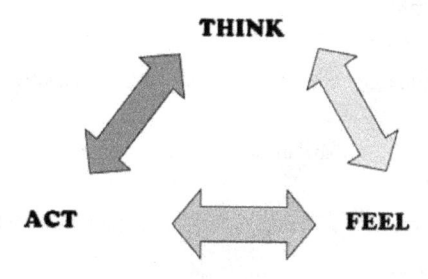

THINK

ACT   **FEEL**

* The word <u>depression</u> is used in many ways. Depression can mean:

  o a <u>feeling</u> that lasts a few minutes

  o a <u>mood</u> that lasts a few hours or a few days

  o a <u>condition</u> that:

  > lasts for at least two weeks
  >
  > causes strong emotional suffering
  >
  > makes it difficult to carry out our daily activities

* People with depression generally have following symptoms:

  feeling sad or down nearly every day

  not being interested in things or unable to enjoy things you used to enjoy

  appetite and/or weight change (eating more or less than you are used to)

  sleeping problems (difficulties falling asleep, waking up often, waking up too early or being unable to fall back asleep, sleeping too much) changes in how fast you move (either being too restless or moving very slow)

feeling tired all the time

feeling worthless or guilty

problems thinking, concentrating, or making decisions

thinking about death or hurting yourself (suicide).

- ❖ Talking about the kind of thoughts they have when they feel sad or depressed:
  - ◦ What kinds of thoughts pass through your mind when you feel depressed or sad?
  - ◦ What do you do when you feel depressed?
  - ◦ How do you get along with others when you are depressed?
  - o How do you get along with others when you are depressed?

"GROUP COUNSELING SESSION - 2"

Objective: To make the participants understand about anxiety.

❖ What is Anxiety?

Anxiety is the feeling we get when our body responds to a frightening or threatening experience. It has been called the fight or flight response. It is simply your body preparing for action either to fight danger or run away from it as fast as possible. The purpose of the physical symptoms of anxiety therefore is to prepare your body to cope with threat. To understand what is happening in your body, imagine that you are about to be attacked. As soon as you are aware of the threat your muscles tense ready for action. Your heard beats faster to carry blood to you muscles and brain, where it is most needed. You breathe faster to provide oxygen which is needed for energy. You sweat to stop your body overheating. Your mouth becomes dry and your stomach may have butterflies.

The fight or flight response is a really basic system that probably goes back to the days of cave men, and is present in animals who depend on it for their survival. Fortunately, nowadays we are not often in such life or death situations, but unfortunately many of the stresses we do face can't be fought or run away from, so the symptoms don't help. In fact they often make us feel worse, especially if we don't understand them.

- **What causes anxiety?**

There are many reasons why someone becomes anxious.

> Some people may have an anxious personality and have learned to worry.
>
> Others may have a series of stressful life events to cope with, for example grief.
>
> Others may be under pressure, at school or at home.

❖ **What keeps anxiety going?**

Thoughts (something awful is going to happen to me)
⇩

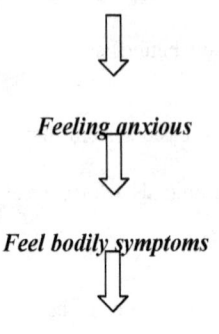

Feeling anxious
⇩

Feel bodily symptoms
⇩

Feeling anxious

Anxiety often becomes a vicious circle where our symptoms, thoughts and behavior keep the anxiety going. a vicious circle where our symptoms, thoughts and behavior keeps the anxiety going.

Students were given anxiety checklist. **Appendix-2**

"GROUP COUNSELING SESSION - 3"

Objective: - Introduction to the concept of "How Our Thoughts Affect Our Mood" (How we feel).

❖ Having certain types of thoughts can make you feel more or less depressed. By "thoughts" we mean "things that we tell ourselves."

❖ Thoughts can have an effect on your body

❖ Thoughts can have an effect on your actions (what you do)

❖ Thoughts can have an effect on your mood (how you feel)

For example: You're walking down a deserted street and you see a person walking quickly behind you. He looks serious, he is looking at you and you think that he is going to mug or rob you. Immediately, your body, your actions and your mood react to this thought. You start sweating, your heart races, and you feel a knot in your stomach. You start looking over your shoulder and walking faster. You feel nervous, afraid. The person reaches you, and quickly walks past you, getting farther and farther away. You think he was just in a hurry.

There are four goals we want to work towards:

1. To lessen or eliminate feelings of depression.
2. To shorten the time you feel depressed.
3. To learn ways to prevent or avoid getting depressed again.

Students were given mood thermometer. (Appendix 3)

"GROUP COUNSELING SESSION - 4"

Objective: - To understand thoughts and types of thought people have.

❖ What are thoughts?

Asking participants about thoughts.

Thoughts are ideas (phrases or sentences) that we tell ourselves. We are constantly talking to ourselves internally, but often we're not always aware of it. It is helpful to think about thoughts as "objects" (ideas) that have a real effect on our bodies and minds.

❖ How do people with depression think?

Of these thoughts you mentioned, which ones have you had?

People with depression tend to have different types of negative thoughts (inflexible, judgmental, destructive and unnecessary). *They were asked to use the contrast between the different types of thoughts.*

Table 3.6

Thoughts	Example
NEGATIVE	Thoughts are all thoughts that make you feel bad, for example: "I am always going to feel depressed" or "I am useless
POSITIVE	Thoughts make you feel better, for example: "I can do things to feel better." "I am getting better each day."
INFLEXIBLE	*Inflexible* thoughts are thoughts that are rigid, thoughts that don't change. For example, a depressed adolescent might think: "I'm the only one they ask to do things at our house." "I can't do anything right."
FLEXIBLE	A *flexible* thought that could help avoid depressed feelings could be: "My parents almost always ask me to do things, but sometimes they ask my sister." "There are lots of times when I do things right."
JUDGMENTAL	*Judgmental* thoughts are negative thoughts about us. For example, a depressed adolescent might think: "I'm ugly" o "I'm a loser".
CONSTRUCTIVE	I can learn to control my life, so I can do what I really want.
UNNECESSARY	*Unnecessary* thoughts don't change anything and they make us feel bad. For example, "A hurricane is going to hit us" or "something bad is going to happen to my parents" or "they're not going to give me permission to go".

❖ How do people who aren't depressed think?

Participants were illustrated the differences between thoughts that depressed people have versus thoughts that people who aren't depressed have.

> They can see the positive side of things
>
> Don't define themselves by their mistakes, they learn from them
>
> They have hope for change

"GROUP COUNSELING SESSION-5"

Objective: - Making participants understand thinking errors.

<u>All or nothing thinking:</u>

This is when you look at things as if they were completely good or completely bad. For example, if you make a mistake doing something, you think all your work was useless. You might think, "I'm not even going to try out for the team because I'll never get picked." Or "I can't do anything right."

<u>Mental Filter</u>:

This is when you take a single negative event and you focus on it in such a way that you see everything as negative and think everything is going wrong. It also refers to making or seeing things as bigger than they really are. For example, "a patient came into treatment one day and told us that she had seen a dead bird on the sidewalk and it made her feel really bad. She had walked through a beautiful garden, full of trees and flowers and all she saw was the dead bird."

Discounting the positive:

This is when you don't notice positive things that happen you only see the negative things. Or you when positive things happen they seem less important to you than they really are. For example, you might believe that nobody likes you to the extent that if someone is nice to you, you think that something must be wrong with that person. Or if someone tells you how good you look, you think he or she says it just so you won't feel bad.

Jumping to the wrong conclusions:

This is when you come to conclusions too quickly and you see the negative side of things. There are two types:

Mind reading:

This is when you assume what someone is thinking without really knowing. For example, you see that someone is angry and you think the person doesn't like you or that the person is angry with you. It might well be that the person is having his/her own difficulties. Other examples: "Dad thinks I'm stupid" or "the coach won't let me play anymore because I didn't score in the game, he thinks I am a bad player."

Fortune-telling:

This is when you feel and predict that only disasters and tragedies will happen to you in the future. For example, "I'm going to flunk out of school" or "I won't have any friends at my new school" or "No one's going to want to dance with me at the party" or "I'm not going to the audition because I'll never be picked."

Taking your feelings too seriously:

This is when you think that your feelings are the only version of reality. For example, you think, "I feel so sad that it proves what a disaster I am" or "I'm so lonely that my life has no meaning." "I am always bored so other people probably seem me as a boring person."

Should/Perfectionism:

This is when you try to motivate yourself with shoulds; that is, with what you believe people should or have to do or say. Even if there are things you need to do, it's important to be careful not to have unrealistic, excessive or inflexible expectations for yourself. For example, you might think, "I should get all As in school" or "My Mom should pay attention to me all the time. It's better to do things the best you can and because you want to, not because you feel guilty. When you think shoulds about other people, you get angry and frustrated if they don't do things the way you expect them to.

Labeling yourself or others:

Only because you make one mistake, you start to think you're a loser. For example, you might say, "I yelled at Mom, I'm a bad daughter" or "I'm stupid because I have bad grades" or "I'm ugly." You might also label others: "The teacher is stupid because she scolded me." "She's a traitor because now she hangs out with other friends besides me."

Blaming oneself:

This is when you blame yourself for the negative things that happen around you and over which you have no control. For example, if something bad happens to one of your family members or friends, you feel as if it was your fault because you couldn't prevent it. Or if your parents get divorced, you feel it was your fault because they were always arguing in front of you.

"GROUP COUNSELING SESSION-6"

Objective: - To make participants aware of how they physically experience emotions.

- Body tracing activity

Students were asked to choose a partner they feel comfortable with as they will be getting in your space. The partner being traced chooses a colored marker, lies down on the tracing paper provided.

The partner completing the tracing should maintain appropriate boundaries and respect their partner's need for safety and comfort.

The partner being traced should think of a time they have experienced anxiety, all while thinking about the shapes, colors, or textures they notice in their body from head to toe. Switch partners once tracing is complete on the first partner.

Once both partners have been traced, each partner colors their emotions inside their body – highlighting where they feel anxiety in their body.

- Then they were asked

    If they were able to identify their physical sensations related to their anxiety?

To what degree they felt the sensation?

Were they able to know in what parts they feel the anxiety?

Referred from :-

Kendall, P., & Hedtke, K. (2006). *Cognitive-behavior therapy for anxious children: therapist manual* (3rd ed.). Ardmore, PA: Workbook Publishing, Inc.

Merrell, K. W. (2001). *Helping students overcome depression and anxiety: A practical guide.* New York, NY: The Guilford Press.

"GROUP COUNSELING SESSION – 7"

Objective: - Decreasing thoughts that make you feel bad

- ❖ Interrupt Your Thoughts

    When a thought is ruining your mood, we can identify it and try to interrupt it. First, identify the thought. Next, tell yourself: "This thought is ruining my mood, so I am going to change it or substitute it for a positive one."

- ❖ Time To Worry

    Set aside "time to worry" each day so that you can concentrate completely on necessary thoughts and leave the rest of the day free of worries. The "time to worry" can be 10 to 30 minutes each day.

- ❖ Laugh at your problems by exaggerating them.

    If you have a good sense of humor, try to laugh at your worries. If you feel you don't have a good sense of humor, try to do it any way you can. Sometimes this can take away the pain of certain hardships.

- ❖ Consider The Worst That Could Happen

    Often some of the fears we have about what could happen make us feel depressed and they paralyze us.

To help you stop making negative predictions and prepare yourself for what could happen, it's useful to ask yourself – What could happen if ____? Or what would really be the worst thing that could happen if_____?

Remember that the worst thing that could happen is only one of many possibilities and just because it's the worst doesn't mean that is the most probable.

It's good to ask yourself whether you're exaggerating what could happen. Maybe none of the things you fear will happen, but if you consider the different possibilities you'll be better prepared.

o An example, you have failing grades in several classes. Your parents are pressuring you and you're afraid of flunking your grade. You could think – what is the worst that could happen if I fail? One possibility is that you'll have to take tutoring or repeat a class during the summer and your parents will be upset. You would feel bad and possibly your parents would be upset for some time, but you could handle it, and resides, you could review the material you didn't learn so well in order to get better grades next year.

"GROUP COUNSELING SESSION-8"

Objective: - Increasing Positive Thoughts

CONGRATULATE YOURSELF

Students were asked to make a statement about a specific area of behavior, beginning with

1. I congratulate myself for ... Things you have done for a friend
2. Work in school
3. How I have earned some money
4. Something I have bought recently
5. How you usually spend your money
6. Habits you have
7. Something you do often
8. What you are proudest of in your life
9. Something you have shared
10. Something you tried hard for
11. Something I done to help someone else

"GROUP COUNSELING SESSION-9"

Objective: - To make participants understand that the Activities That We Do Affect our Mood.

- ❖ Through our activities we can tell how we feel.

    The fewer pleasant activities people do, the more depressed they feel.

    Do you stop doing things because you feel depressed? or Do you feel depressed because you stop doing things?

    The most probable answer is **BOTH**:

The fewer things you do, the more depressed you feel. The more depressed you feel, the fewer things you do. This is called a "VICIOUS CYCLE."

Figure 3.2

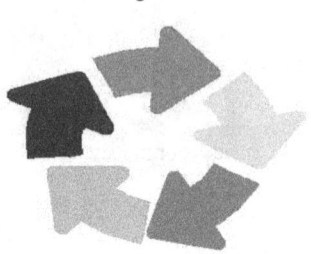

To break the vicious cycle you can increase those activities that make you feel better.

These activities can be called "pleasant", "encouraging", "inspiring", etc. We call them "pleasant."

Pleasant activities need not to be something special they can be your regular activities (like watching tv,music,playing,reading,internet surfing etc.) or you can try something special too .(like going for a movie, helping someone, travel etc) .

Sometimes obstacles get in the way of our doing certain pleasant activities.

- ❖ Your Thoughts

    - What kind of thoughts helps you enjoy an activity?
    - What thoughts make it hard for you to enjoy an activity?
    - Have you ever enjoyed an activity that you thought you wouldn't?

Appendix - 4

"GROUP COUNSELING SESSION-10"

Objective: - To make participants understand how to make realistic goals.

Question asked to the participants.

- ❖ WHAT ARE GOALS?

    How can reaching goals help you feel better?

- ❖ TYPES OF GOALS:

    Short term goals

    Things you'd like to do soon (say in the one month)

    Long Term Goals

    Things you'd like to do at some point in your life

- ❖ IDENTIFYING GOALS – WHAT ARE YOUR GOALS?

    Asking the participants to write down their short term, long term goals on the worksheet of Personal Goals. **(Appendix 5)**

- ❖ SETTING CLEAR, CONCRETE GOALS:

Set clear, concrete goals so that you can be sure of when you've reached them.

Table 3.7

UNCLEAR GOALS (global - general)	CLEAR GOALS (specific - concrete)
Be less bored	Go to the mall once a week
Be a good friend	Spend three hours a week doing pleasant things with your friends
Be a good musician	Spend x hours a week practicing an instrument
Get better grades	Study for two hours every afternoon
Lose weight	Walk 30 minutes a day and follow a healthy diet (portions, healthy foods, 10% less calories, or most appropriate)

Which one of your goals can be clearer and more concrete?

- ❖ BREAK DOWN YOUR BIG GOALS INTO SMALLER PARTS:

  Make sure that each part can be achieved without too much effort. If your goal is to be a good baseball player, then you could start by finding out were the nearest baseball park is and what times you can practice.

  Which one of your goals could you divide into smaller parts?

- ❖ SETTING REALISTIC GOALS

  It is often difficult to determine beforehand what's realistic and what's not. What's not realistic today can be realistic in the future. However, if you find you can't meet most of your goals now, then they are probably not realistic for you at this time.

"GROUP COUNSELING SESSION-11"

Objective: - To make participants understand how to achieve their goals

- ❖ What are some of the obstacles that prevent you from achieving your goals?

  Asking participants about what are the obstacles for them.

- ❖ To make changes in our lives, sometimes we need to make changes in our goals.

- ❖ Things that are realistic might become unrealistic.

  For example: An adolescent plays volleyball and she'd like to play in a major league. She hurts her knee badly during a game, and she can't keep playing that sport. However, maybe she can become a volleyball coach or assistant coach.

- ❖ Things that were unrealistic might become realistic.

    For example: An adolescent wanted to be able to drive his mother's car. His mother told him that he still wasn't old enough to do so. He felt like he would never get to drive, he saw it as so far away. Finally he turned 18 and his mom let him drive under her supervision. *Asking students if they have somethimg like this in their mind..* If a change occurs in your life that requires a change in goals, then maybe you'll have to:

    Enjoy activities in new ways

    Develop new interests, abilities and activities.

    Establish realistic goals.

    Recognize the positive things you do to reach them.

    Congratulate and reward yourself mentally and in real life.

"GROUP COUNSELING SESSION-12"

Objective: - To make participants understand the importance of social support

The support we receive from being in contact with other people is important for our health. -- The contacts we have with our family and friends create a kind of protective social network or "social support network".

The system or "social support network" refers to people who are close to us and with whom you share important information or important moments of your life. These people can be family, friends, neighbors, classmates and acquaintances. In general, the stronger the social support we receive, the more we are able to confront difficult situations.

- ❖ What is your social support network like?

    Who are your friends? How often do you see them? What do you do? Who do you trust? Exercise: Recreate your social support network using the diagram on the **My Social Support Network** worksheet. **(Appendix-6)**

- ❖ Two important principles to keep in mind in the future.

    If your social support network is too small, make it larger. Your network is too small if there is no one you trust to talk about your personal matters, if you have no one to go to if you need help, or if you have no friends or acquaintances to do things with.

    If your network is adequate and of a good size, appreciate it and try to keep it strong. In other words, don't let disagreements cause separations between you and the people in your network. Frequent communication helps maintain friendships.

- ❖ Keeping your social support network healthy

Contact with others is very important, be it by phone or in person (talk, listen, go out, do activities together).

Some thoughts that can block this. For example:

"They haven't called me; it looks like they don't care about me."

"They don't like me."

"No one in my family understands me."

"My mom never listens."

"GROUP COUNSELING SESSION-13"

Objective: -How to build better relations/friendships

- ❖ Meeting People

    How do you make friends? What have your friends done to get closer to you? What does a friendly or sociable person do?

    The easiest way to meet other people is by doing an activity you like in the company of others.

    -When you enjoy something, it's more likely that you'll be in a good mood and that way it'll be easier to be sociable and friendly.

    -Even if you don't find anyone in particular that you want to get to know better, you'll be doing something you enjoy and you won't feel it was a waste of your time.

    Since the main focus will be on the activity and not on meeting other people, it's more likely that you'll feel less pressure than you'd feel if the only purpose was meeting new people. If there were people you want to get to know better, it's more probable that they'll have things in common with you.

- ❖ How To Establish And Maintain Healthy Relationships: Being Assertive.

    What's the difference between being passive, assertive and aggressive?

There are three ways we can act and communicate with others:

Being passive means not expressing your feelings to others because you think they'll be annoyed, feel bad or because they are superior to you. You might feel you have to "swallow" your feelings or you'll be rejected.

Being aggressive means treating others with hostility, anger and being insensitive to other people's needs and feelings because you feel yours are more important.

Being assertive means being able to say positive and negative things without feeling bad. You don't always have to say what you think, but it's important to feel that you have that option. You can say things in a nice way that can help resolve situations and maintain the relationship healthy.

"GROUP COUNSELING SESSION 14"

Objective: - Making participants understand the Anxiety Hierarchy.

As confronting social situations can sometimes be a daunting thought, it can be helpful to do so in a gradual way. Creating an exposure hierarchy can help you to do this. An exposure hierarchy is basically a list of social situations which would cause you varying degrees of anxiety The idea is that you confront the easiest (or least anxiety provoking) item on your hierarchy to begin with and work your way through to more difficult items as your confidence grows.

To help you get ideas for your hierarchy, it may help to consider all the social situations and scenarios that:

Make you anxious

You avoid or escape from

You only confront if you are using a 'safety behavior'

It is important that the items on your list cause you varying degrees of anxiety (e.g. speaking to a small group of friends versus a group of work colleagues).

Ranking your hierarchy once you have a list of items for your hierarchy, the next stage is to try to rank them in order of least anxiety provoking to most anxiety provoking. To help, try to predict how anxious you believe each item would make you feel on a scale from 0 to 100, where 100 is the most anxious you have ever felt and 0 is the most relaxed you have ever felt

Once you have completed this, rearrange the items on your list from least anxiety provoking to most anxiety provoking

Confronting the first item on your hierarchy Once you have finalized your hierarchy, the next step is to confront the first item on it as soon as possible

This should be the item that you predict will cause you the least amount of anxiety from your list. During exposure tasks it is important to: Remember that although your anxiety will initially rise during an exposure task-

> It will fall if you remain in the situation for long enough. Be aware that anxiety is a natural and healthy reaction that everyone experiences
> Although it can feel unpleasant, it is not dangerous and will gradually pass if you remain in the situation for long enough. Try to remain in the situation until your anxiety reduces by at least half.

Remember that the more often you expose yourself to an item on your hierarchy, the quicker you will overcome your fear towards it.

Moving onto the next item on your hierarchy once you have overcome your fear towards the first item on your hierarchy, you should follow the same steps with the next item on your hierarchy. Continue through your hierarchy in this manner until you have reached the top and feel more confident about social situations. Remember that as you progress through each stage of your hierarchy your confidence will grow.

"GROUP COUNSELING SESSION 15"

Objective: - Understanding you and your relationship.

In this session we are going to explore how your thoughts, actions and feelings influence your relationships and how your relationships affect these three areas. Before talking about how these three areas are affected by your relationships, it's important to evaluate first how they are when you are alone.

- ❖ BEING ALONE.

    When you're alone, what are your _____ like?

    - thoughts
    - actions or behavior
    - feelings

- ❖ BEING WITH OTHERS YOUR THOUGHTS

    What thoughts do you have when you are with other people?

    Thoughts that prevent you from making friends.

    Thoughts that help you feel comfortable with other people.

    One way to feel better is to shift the focus of attention from you to the other person and think about how he/she feels. Think about how you feel when you're going to meet new people. Other people probably feel the same way.

- ❖ YOUR EXPECTATIONS

    What can you expect from other people?

What can others expect from you?

If your expectations are too high, you'll be disappointed and maybe you'll become frustrated.

If your expectations are too low, you won't expect anything from the relationship and you might lose the chance to develop good relationships. Also, if you expect little from people, you're not giving them the chance to show you what they can really offer.

❖ YOUR ACTIONS/BEHAVIOR

How do you approach others?

What impression do you think you give off to others?

- Your face: Do you smile often? Do you make eye contact?
- Your body: Do you look tired or worn out?

- Your appearance: Is it appropriate for the time and place?

- Your speech: Is it too slow or too soft to hear you? Do you speak with anger or irritation? Do you raise your voice?

- Your conversation: Do you show interest in what other people say, or do you ignore or criticize them?

- Your attitude: Do you complain a lot? Are you in a bad mood? Do you offend others with your attitude?

❖ YOUR FEELINGS

How do your feelings affect your relationships?

Different emotions can influence the way you relate to others. There are times when we experience negative emotions (i.e. anger, sadness) that have nothing to do with the person we're relating to. However, we let these feelings affect the relationship. This is way it's important to be able to identify and manage our feelings in a healthy way.

What feelings do you have when you're with others?

- ❖ Identifying our feelings when we're with other people can help us evaluate the quality of our relationship.

- ❖ For this, it's important to:

   Recognize how your feel and why you're feeling that way

   Communicate in an assertive or appropriate way what you feel

   The difference between being passive, assertive or aggressive:

Assertiveness = is being able to share positive and negative feelings clearly and comfortably (even if you think the other person won't like what you're saying). Changing your point of view can help you to be more assertive instead of being passive. For example, if you frequently think, "I don't want to make anyone feel bad," try to think, "Saying what I think can help us communicate better and resolve the situation. At least I can let people know what I think."

"GROUP COUNSELING SESSION 16"

Objective: - To develop certain Communication skills.

- ❖ Active listening

    When you are talking to someone, listen to what they are saying instead of thinking about you are going to say back or respond. If you're thinking about what you're going to answer, you might miss part of what the person is telling you. People often argue about what somebody said without knowing if that was what the person really wanted to say or express.

- ❖ To improve your active listening and communication skills:

    -Repeat what the other person said in your own words so you can be sure you understood him/her correctly. For example, "I understand that you're saying_____."

    - Ask the person directly what he/she meant to say. For example, What did you mean by _____?"

    - When we become mad with someone, instead of attacking them, it's more effective to say what you think and/or feel in relation to what they are doing, or their actions.

    Instead of saying – "You (are/always/never)..." It's better to say – "I feel _____/I think_____." When we attack people they generally become defensive and aren't going to listen to what we really want to tell them.

- ❖ Examples of verbalizations where you attack the other person: "You're unfair." "You never do what I want."

- Alternatives: "When you scold me before listening to what I have to say, I feel frustrated." "When you say no, I feel like you don't care about me and don't want me to have any fun." "I feel that you're not listening."
- Find the right moment to talk. The best times aren't when the person is doing something, or there isn't enough time to talk or if you're in the middle of an argument.
- Consider your non-verbal language (gestures, facial expressions, posture, etc.) Non-verbal language is 80% of communication.
- Consider the tone of your voice.

    Follow the example of assertive people you know and ask them for suggestions (i.e., family, friends, and teachers).

    You can decide to change.

- *Before* being with other people

    Thinking differently: To change your feelings towards others, you can decide beforehand the kind of thoughts you want to have when you're with them.

    Acting differently: If you want to change your behavior when you're with others, decide beforehand how you would like to act when you are around them.

DAY 16: "GROUP COUNSELING SESSION 17"

Objective- Making participants understand How Breathing affects Feelings.

The way we breathe is strongly linked to the way we feel. When we are relaxed we breathe slowly, and when we are anxious we breathe more quickly.

- <u>Normal breathing</u>

When we breathe we take in oxygen (O2) that is used by the body. This process creates carbon dioxide (CO2), a waste product that we breathe out. When our breathing is relaxed the levels of oxygen and carbon dioxide are balanced - this allows our body to function evidently.

Figure 3.3

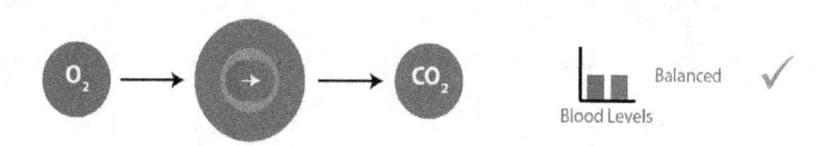

❖ Exercise breathing

Our breathing rate increases during exercise to take in more oxygen. The body uses the extra oxygen to fuel the muscles and so produces more carbon dioxide. The increased breathing rate leads to more carbon dioxide being expelled. This means that the balance between oxygen and carbon dioxide levels is maintained.

Figure 3.4

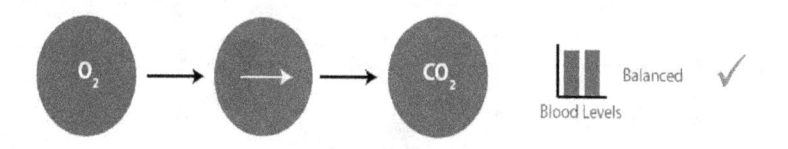

❖ Anxious breathing

When we are anxious our breathing rate increases: we take in more oxygen and breathe out more carbon dioxide than usual. However, because the body is not working any harder than normal it is not using up any extra oxygen, and so it is not producing any extra carbon dioxide. Because carbon dioxide is being expelled faster than it is being produced its concentration in the blood goes down (leading to a temporary change in the pH of the blood called respiratory alkalosis). This change in CO2 blood concentration can lead us to feeling unpleasantly lightheaded, tingly in our -fingers and toes, clammy, and sweaty.

When our breathing returns to its usual rate the levels of carbon dioxide in the blood return to normal, and the symptoms resolve. You can deliberately relax your breathing to feel better.

Figure 3.5

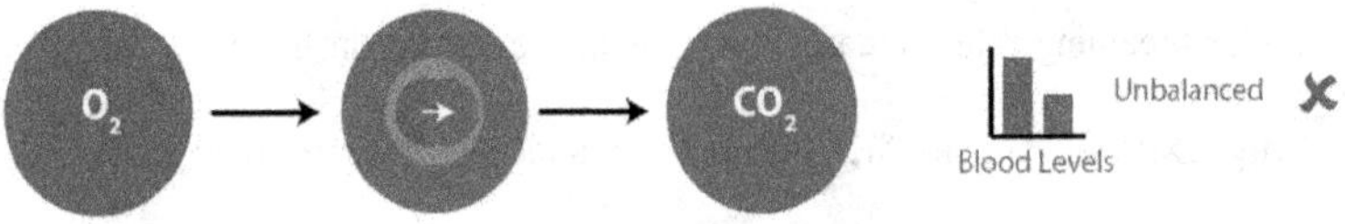

Relaxed Breathing

When we are anxious or threatened our breathing speeds up in order to get our body ready for danger. Relaxed breathing (sometimes called abdominal or diaphragmatic breathing) signals the body that it is safe to relax. Relaxed breathing is *slower* and *deeper* than normal breathing, and it happens lower in the body (the belly rather than the chest).

```
In-breath        Pause         Out-breath       Pause
1 ... 2 ... 3 ... 4    1 ...        1 ... 2 ... 3 ... 4    1 ...
```

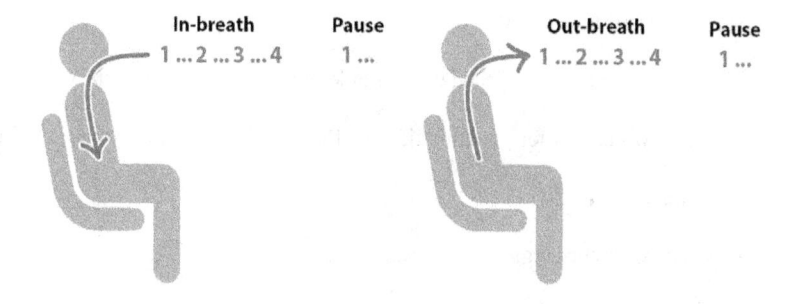

How to do relaxed breathing

- To practice make sure you are sitting or lying comfortably
- Close your eyes if you are comfortable doing so
- Try to breathe through your nose rather than your mouth
- Deliberately slow your breathing down. Breathe in to a count of 4, pause for a moment, then breathe out to a count of four
- Make sure that your breaths are *smooth*, *steady*, and *continuous* - not jerky
- Pay particular attention to your out-breath - make sure it is smooth and steady

Am I doing it right? What should I be paying attention to?

- Relaxed breathing should be low down in the abdomen (belly), and not high in the chest. You can check this by putting one hand on your stomach and one on your chest. Try to keep the top hand still, your breathing should only move the bottom hand.
- Focus your attention on your breath - some people find it helpful to count in their head to begin with (*"In ... two ... three ... four ... pause ... Out ... two ... three ... four... pause ..."*)

How long and how often?

- Try breathing in a relaxed way for at least a few minutes at a time - it might take a few minutes for you to notice an effect. If you are comfortable, aim for 5-10 minutes
- Try to practice regularly - perhaps three times a day

Variations and troubleshooting

- Find a slow breathing rhythm that is comfortable for you. Counting to 4 isn't an absolute rule. Try 3 or 5. The important thing is that the breathing is slow and steady
- Some people find the sensation of relaxing to be unusual or uncomfortable at first . But this normally passes with practice. Do persist and keep practicing.

"GROUP COUNSELING SESSION 18"

Objective: - Introducing the concept of mindfulness to participants.

MINDFULNESS

Being mindful means that you are paying attention to, and therefore living in, the present moment. Most of the time, our minds are reaching forward to the future, and we often start to worry about things that are unknown. This raises our anxiety level. Or our minds are reaching back into the past, and we may feel guilt or regret about something we have done or said. This raises our anxiety level, too.

Being mindful means being non-judgemental and accepting about whatever is happening in the present moment. Focusing on the present moment can help you let go of anxiety.

Practicing mindfulness can decrease you anxiety as well as enrich your life experiences because you are more fully present in everything that you do.

Using some type of food, participants were asked to eat this food slowly while practicing to focus on the present. Instruct the group to use all five senses to experience the activity. Participants were asked to pay close attention to exactly what they are seeing, hearing, feeling, smelling, and tasting as they do this.

Participants were advised that whenever they notice themselves feeling anxious it is because they have moved their thinking into the future or the past.

They were reminded that when their mind wanders away to bring it back to what they are doing in the present moment.

Referred from :-

Schab, L. (2005). *The anxiety workbook for teens.* Norwalk, CT: Instant Help Publications.

'GROUP COUNSELING SESSION 19"

Objective; - How to stop negative thoughts.

When we feel nervous we can take a break and mentally give ourselves a time out. Let your mind relax and take a deep breath. Pay attention to your body's natural ability to relax and feel at peace. Feeling at peace can give you energy.

❖ Progressive Muscle Relaxation

1. Breathe deeply 3 times, slowly exhaling after each breath. When you exhale imagine that the tension in your body is slowly beginning to disappear.

2. Close your hand into a fist. Hold it for 7 seconds; now let it go for 15 seconds... Feel the tension... Now let go of the fist and open your hand...Feel the tension disappear. Now your hand feels heavy...

3. Tense your forearm as if you were showing off your muscles in both arms. Hold it....and release.

4. Tense your triceps extending your arms in front of your body. Hold...and release...Feel the tension decrease and disappear.

5. Tense the muscles in your forehead by raising your eyebrows as much as you can...Hold....and release...Picture your muscles as becoming soft and relaxed...

6. Tense the muscles around your eyes by squeezing them shut...Hold... and relax...Feel a sense of deep relaxation spreading out all over that area...

7. Tense your jaw by opening your mouth real wide until you stretch those muscles...Hold...and release...Let your jaw drop...

8. Tense the muscles in the back of you neck as if you were going to touch your back with your head. Focus only on tensing the muscles in your neck...Hold...and release...

9. Tense the muscles in your shoulders raising them as if you were going to touch your ears with them...Hold...and release...

10. Tense the muscles in your chest by inhaling deeply...Hold it...and exhale slowly...Imagine all the tension in your chest is slowly disappearing as you exhale...

11. Tense the muscles in your abdomen or stomach as if you were to touch your belly button to your back...Hold...and relax. Imagine a wave a relaxation spreading across your stomach.

12. Tense your muscles in your knee...Hold...and release...Feel as your muscles are stretched and completely relaxed.
13. Tense the muscles in your legs slowly pointing your toes towards you...Hold ...and release.
14. Now you're going to do the opposite, pointing your toes in front of you...Hold...and release...
15 Imagine a wave of relaxation is slowly spreading throughout your body...starting at your head and gradually penetrating each group of muscles until it reaches your feet...eliminating any residual tension...

"GROUP COUNSELING SESSION 20"

Objective: - Making participants understand perception and healthy management of reality.

Participants were presented pictures and asked what they see? These pictures were illusion creating and could be interpreted in different ways. ***Appendix-7***

This exercise was to make them understand how our perception about the same thing or event can be different from the others.

- ❖ WE LIVE IN TWO WORLDS:

1) The objective world (the world outside, everything outside of us)
    For example, the places, people and events around us that we can't change (where we live, the school we go to, who are parents are).

2) The subjective (internal) world (our internal world, what's inside our minds) for example, our thoughts, beliefs, wishes, feelings and dreams (how we perceive what we do and what happens to us).

❖ THESE TWO WORLDS ARE OUR REALITY.

The key to feeling emotionally healthy is to learn how to manage these two parts of our reality.

- The objective world, generally speaking, we can't change, but we can learn ways to manage it in a way that it doesn't' affect how we feel so much.
- On the other hand, we can have more control over our subjective world. When people are depressed, the often perceive their subjective world as the only reality.
- When people are depressed they feel that have no control, that there's nothing they can do to feel better. However, things can always change and improve.

❖ ALTERNATIVES

Sometimes we find ourselves in situations in which it's hard to make decisions because we don't see alternatives or we only see one. It can also happen that we feel we don't have any alternatives when things don't happen the way we want them to. On these occasions it helps to consider all the alternatives and not to focus on that fact that you don't have what you really wanted.

The more alternatives you have, the more freedom you'll have.

"GROUP COUNSELING SESSION 21"

Objective: - Termination of the Program

Students were asked about their overall experience.

They were asked about the things they will continue and things they liked the most. They were given the feedback forms to fill in.**Appendix-8**

Heartfelt thanks were given by the counselor to all the students.

Phase 3: POST INTERVENTION PHASE

Post tests were administered on both experimental and control group to measure depression, anxiety, optimism and rumination. All the participants were thanked for their presence and cooperation during the intervention. After collecting the post test scores, data was subjected to statistical analysis.

STATISTICAL ANALYSIS

Descriptive statistics of both the groups and all variables were calculated to compare the pre and post test scores.

t- test was employed to investigate the comparisons in both cases of between and in groups.